Nursing Science

MAJOR PARADIGMS, THEORIES, AND CRITIQUES

Rosemarie Rizzo Parse, R.N., Ph.D.

Professor of Nursing, Graduate Nursing Program
Hunter College of The City University of New York
New York, New York

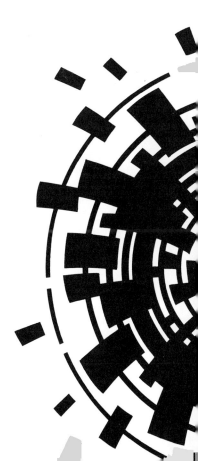

W.B. SAUNDERS COMPANY
Philadelphia o London o Toronto o Mexico City
Rio de Janeiro o Sydney o Tokyo o Hong Kong

W. B. SAUNDERS COMPANY
Harcourt Brace Jovanovich, Inc.

The Curtis Center
Independence Square West
Philadelphia, PA 19106

Library of Congress Cataloging-in-Publication Data

Nursing science.

    1. Nursing—Philosophy. I. Parse, Rosemarie
Rizzo. [DNLM: 1. Nursing. 2. Philosophy, Nursing.
WY 86 N9737]
RT84.5.N878 1987   610.73   86-21904
ISBN 0-7216-1803-0

Editor: Dudley Kay
Designer: Bill Donnelly
Production Manager: Pete Faber
Manuscript Editor: Renee Munoz
Illustration Coordinator: Walt Verbitski
Indexer: Nancy Weaver & Nelle Garrecht

Nursing Science: Major Paradigms, Theories and Critiques ISBN 0-7216-1803-0

Last digit is the print number: 9   8   7   6   5

When a new discovery is reported to the scientific world, they say first, "It is probably not true." When the truth of the proposition has been demonstrated beyond question, they say, "It may be true, but it is not important." When sufficient time has elapsed to fully evidence its importance they say, "Surely it is important, but it is no longer new."

MONTAIGNE

Preface

Paradigm development is an important cornerstone to the foundation of the science of nursing and to the elaboration of its process. The nursing theories comprising each of two paradigms are presented herein: first by the theorists themselves, and then through an evaluation of each theory, based on criteria developed from experts in theory development. Each theory is examined for its structure, correspondence, coherence, and pragmatics.

This volume aims to provide an understanding of nursing science through an examination of paradigmatic perspectives. By using this orientation, attention is focused on the belief systems of the discipline that guide research and practice.

That there are two paradigms—the totality paradigm, the oldest and most dominant view, and the newer simultaneity paradigm—is important for nursing's development as a science. Disciplines develop through the expansion of new knowledge guided by paradigmatic perspectives. These two paradigms embrace very different views of Man and health, and thus create broader and richer options for research and practice.

The chapters are organized to assist the reader in gaining an understanding of the evolution of nursing science. Chapter 1 discusses the meaning and importance of paradigms for scientific disciplines, nursing paradigms and their evolution, and criteria for evaluation of the theories within the paradigms. Chapter 2 develops the emergence of nursing science from a historical perspective, including an examination of nursing science in light of the scientific criteria. The first section overview offers a general view of the totality paradigm. Chapters 3 through 8 set forth different theories of the totality paradigm and critiques of each. The second section overview offers a synopsis of the simultaneity paradigm; Chapters 9 through 12 set forth the theories of the simultaneity paradigm and their critiques.

This book has been written for those nurses interested in nursing theory and its impact on the evolution of nursing science. It is an important reference for those professional nurses who wish to know more about the elements of the extant theories and those who wish to analyze those theories for a better understanding of the process of theory building. Thus this material is most valuable for master's and doctoral degree students who, as developing scholars, are coming to know the discipline of nursing. It is also very valuable for nursing faculty and administrators in universities and major health care settings.

The emergence of a scientific discipline represents an ongoing process that requires specification of the paradigms through creative conceptualization and critical appraisal. This work contributes to the specification of nursing as a scientific discipline through presentation of both creative conceptualizations and critical appraisals.

ROSEMARIE RIZZO PARSE

Contributors

MARY H. HUCH, Ph.D., R.N.
Associate Professor of Nursing, University of Southern Mississippi, Hattiesburg, Mississippi

IMOGENE M. KING, Ed.D., R.N.
Professor of Nursing, University of South Florida, Tampa, Florida

SHARON J. MAGAN, Ph.D., R.N.
Clinical Nurse Specialist, Veterans Administration Medical Center, Pittsburgh, Pennsylvania

DOROTHEA E. OREM, M.S.N.Ed., R.N.
President, Orem and Shields, Nursing Consultants, Savannah, Georgia

HILDEGARD E. PEPLAU, Ed.D., R.N.
Professor of Nursing Emerita, Rutgers University, New Jersey

JOHN R. PHILLIPS, Ph.D., R.N.
Associate Professor of Nursing, New York University, New York, New York

MARTHA E. ROGERS, Sc.D., R.N., F.A.A.N.
Professor Emerita, Division of Nursing, New York University, New York, New York

SR. CALLISTA ROY, Ph.D., R.N., F.A.A.N.
Professor of Nursing, Mount Saint Mary's College, Los Angeles, California; Associate Research Nurse, University of California at San Francisco

MARY JANE SMITH, Ph.D., R.N.
Professor of Nursing, West Virginia University, Morgantown, West Virginia

ANN L. WHALL, Ph.D., R.N.
Professor of Nursing, University of Michigan, Detroit, Michigan

Contents

1

Paradigms and Theories

ROSEMARIE RIZZO PARSE

Nursing is a scientific discipline. Consistent with other disciplines, it encompasses more than one paradigm to guide inquiry toward an understanding of Man and health. The two major paradigms identified in nursing are the Man-environment totality paradigm and the Man-environment simultaneity paradigm (Parse and others, 1985). Before presenting an explanation of these nursing paradigms, it is important to specify the meaning of paradigms in scientific disciplines.

1

Paradigms of a Scientific Discipline

A scientific discipline is a body of knowledge that encompasses more than one paradigm to guide inquiry toward an understanding of phenomena. A paradigm is a worldview about the phenomena of concern in a discipline (Kuhn, 1970). It guides inquiry and thus creates scientific development. A worldview arises from new conceptualizations as the scientists in a discipline forge the way to different understandings of phenomena. The emergence of a paradigm occurs when scientists venture outside the primary operating belief system to explain, describe, or predict a situation involving the phenomena of a discipline. As the different conceptualizations become more specified and the beliefs more explicit, the paradigm grows and is recognized as a competing view; thus a paradigm shift is evident. Paradigm development is necessary for the enhancement of a discipline, and each one gives rise to several theories. Theories are grounded in the belief system of the paradigm, which means that the definitions of the concepts of the theories are congruent with beliefs set forth in the paradigm. Theories of a paradigm are the specific tools that guide practice and research.

A theory is a set of interrelated concepts at the same level of discourse that explains, describes, or makes predictions about the phenomena of a discipline. It includes in its overall structure assumptions, principles, concepts, and propositions—the basic elements of a theory. An *assumption* is a statement about the phenomena central to the discipline that represents the beliefs the theorist holds true. The assumptions underpin the theoretical conceptualization and are written at the philosophical level of discourse. The philosophical level of discourse is formulated at the highest level of abstraction followed in descending order by theoretical and empirical levels of abstraction. An idea can be presented at the philosophical, theoretical, and empirical levels; at each lower level the language of discourse becomes more concrete. A *concept* is an abstract idea written at the theoretical level of discourse and is a building block of a theory. A *principle* is a statement explaining an idea by joining two or more concepts written at the theoretical level. A *proposition* is a statement that relates two or more concepts from a principle in a way that guides research and practice. The proposition moves concepts from the theoretical to the empirical level of discourse.

A theory, then, contains a clear, concise description of the phenomena of the discipline and well-defined principles and propositions using language that specifies the concepts at a common level of discourse. A theory is based on conceptually congruent philosophical assumptions. It is written at an abstract level and requires the construction of congruent, empirically stated propositions for testing in research and practice. The purpose of a theory in scientific disciplines is to guide research to enhance the science by supporting existing knowledge or generating new knowledge. The development of a science, then, occurs within the contexts of the paradigms.

Nursing As a Scientific Discipline

Nursing's emergence as a science is clear: it has moved from a vocation to a discipline with competing paradigms. The phenomena of concern to nursing are Man and health, first identified as nursing's major concern by Nightingale (1859), about one hundred and twenty-five years ago.

Two major ways of viewing Man and health have evolved over time. Nurse leaders such as Peplau (1952), Henderson (1955), Orlando (1961), Hall (1966), Levine (1973), and Johnson (1980) guided the early development of the discipline. More recently, in the past 15 years, Orem (1985), Roy (1976, 1981, 1984), King (1981), Rogers (1970, 1980), and Parse (1981) have set forth systematized theoretical structures grounded in views of Man and health that specify the substance of the discipline. The views about Man and health in these systematized structures fall naturally into two specific paradigms, the totality paradigm and the simultaneity paradigm (Parse and others, 1985).

Nursing Paradigms

The names of the nursing paradigms reflect the inherent beliefs about Man and health, the phenomena of concern to nursing. The Man-environment totality paradigm posits Man as a total, summative organism whose nature is a combination of bio-psycho-social-spiritual features. This worldview specifies the environment as the internal and external stimuli surrounding Man. Man adapts to and interacts with the environment to maintain balance and achieve goals. This belief is very different from the belief that Man is a unitary being in continuous mutual interrelationship with the environment, and whose health is a negentropic unfolding, which is the view set forth in the simultaneity paradigm.

The predominant paradigm in nursing has been and continues to be the totality paradigm. Nursing's evolution is rooted in a belief system congruent with the view of Man as a mechanistic organism who adapts to the environment and strives toward a state of well-being. Nursing's emergence as a natural science alongside medicine crystallized this view. The totality paradigm as the primary operating belief system permeated the works of the early developers of nursing science mentioned above, as well as the works of Roy (1976, 1981, 1984), Orem (1985), and King (1981), who set forth more systematized structures.

In 1970 Rogers posited the first view of nursing outside this primary operating belief system, when she posited Man as more than and different from the sum of parts, changing mutually and simultaneously with the environment (Rogers, 1970). This view, which she further developed and which was elaborated by Parse (1981), is now recognized as an alternative view, called the simultaneity paradigm. This alternative view provides the theoretical grounding for research and practice, focusing on Man as a freely choosing being cocreating health through mutual interchange with the environment (Parse and others, 1985). The emergence of different nursing paradigms and congruent theories advances the boundaries of the discipline and thus is necessary for the development of nursing science.

Evaluation of Theories and Frameworks

One aspect inherent in the enhancement of a discipline is the critique of the scholarly works of that discipline. The scholarly works of a discipline set forth the theories of a paradigm that guide research and practice. Critical appraisal of the body of knowledge of any discipline promotes the expansion and specification of that discipline and is a way of teaching aspiring scholars the components of the knowledge base and the process of theory building.

Critical appraisal of frameworks and theories is a systematic process of evaluating extant works in light of established norms. Many such norms have been explicitly set forth in nursing over the past 20 years (Chinn and Jacobs, 1983; Duffey and Muhlenkamp, 1974; Hardy, 1974; Ellis, 1968; Fawcett, 1984; Fitzpatrick and Whall, 1983; Stevens, 1984; Meleis, 1985). These norms relate to semantics, logical consistency, simplicity, aesthetics, and pragmatics, all of which evolved in some way from Kaplan (1964), who established norms for validation of theories. He wrote that "norms of validation can be grouped according to the three major philosophical conceptions of truth: correspondence or semantical norms, coherence or syntactical norms and pragmatic or functional norms" (Kaplan, 1964, p. 312).

Judging a theory as valid does not mean that all scientists in a field find the theory useful. Rather, a valid theory is one worth publishing, teaching, and using (Kaplan, 1964). The critique criteria utilized for this work were constructed utilizing the work of Kaplan (1964). The two major areas of the critique framework are structure and process criteria; full delineation of the evaluative criteria is shown in Table 1-1.

STRUCTURE CRITERIA

Structure criteria are those elements that refer to the physiognomy of the theory. Criteria related to the basic structure of a theory elaborate the historical evolution, demonstrate the presence of the essential elements, and show definitions and relationships of

TABLE 1
Criteria for Evaluation of Nursing Theories

Structure Criteria Questions
1. How is the historical evolution of the theory described?
2. Are the philosophical assumptions underpinning the theory explicitly stated?
3. Are the principles, concepts, and propositions of the theory explicitly stated?
4. How is Man defined in the theory?
5. How is health defined in the theory?
6. Does the theory explicate the relationship between Man and health?

Process Criteria Questions
Correspondence
1. Does the theory fit with the established general knowledge about Man and health?
2. Does the theory interrelate concepts at the same level of discourse to describe, explain, or predict about Man and health?
3. With what paradigmatic perspective does the theory correspond?
4. Does the theory correspond with the philosophical assumptions?
5. Are the principles, concepts, and propositions described parsimoniously in abstract terms?
6. Is the meaning of the principles, concepts, and propositions clear?
7. Is the meaning of each concept of the theory at a consistent level of discourse?

Coherence
1. How do the principles of the theory relate to other theories?
2. Is there a logical flow from philosophical assumptions to propositions?
3. Is the theory structured in a symmetrically aesthetic way?

Pragmatics
1. Can the theory be moved down the ladder of abstraction for use in research and practice?
2. Does the theory generate research questions for investigation?
3. Does the theory offer guidelines for practice?
4. Is there evidence of support for the theory in research and practice?
5. How can the contribution of the theory to nursing science be described?

the phenomena of concern in the discipline. Primarily these criteria provide a framework to uncover the historical grounding of the theory and to judge whether the essential elements are present.

The following are the specific questions related to the structure criteria used in this work to critique the theories presented in this volume:

1. How is the historical evolution of the theory described?

2. Are the philosophical assumptions underpinning the theory explicitly stated?

3. Are the principles, concepts, and propositions of the theory explicitly stated?

4. How is Man defined in the theory?

5. How is health defined in the theory?

6. Does the theory explicate the relationship between Man and health?

PROCESS CRITERIA

Process criteria are correspondence, coherence, and pragmatics. The meaning of these criteria emerges from Kaplan (1964).

Correspondence

Correspondence refers to the semantic integrity of the theory. Semantic integrity is essential to the validation of a theory in that it refers to the consistency of meanings among the terms used to explain the theory and how these meanings relate to the established general knowledge about the phenomena of concern in the discipline. Semantic integrity is revealed through substance and clarity. Substance refers to the soundness of the meaning of the principles, concepts, and propositions and their relationship to existing knowledge, and clarity refers to the sharpness of meaning expressed in the definitions of the terms themselves. A measure of correspondence is how well the theory fits with one paradigm or the other in the discipline of nursing.

Beliefs about Man and health are set forth as the assumptions underpinning a theory. It is important that the expressed meanings of each of the concepts in the theory are consistent with the meanings set forth in the philosophical assumptions. This enhances substance and demonstrates an aspect of semantic integrity. To further demonstrate semantic integrity, there must be clarity and consistency in the definitions of the principles, concepts, and propositions themselves. The meaning of the concepts within a theory should be expressed at a consistent level of discourse. This means that the concepts joined to form the propositions are stated at a similar level of abstraction (Kim, 1983; Walker and Avant, 1983). To mix levels of abstraction in a theory blurs its meaning and violates the criterion of correspondence.

Correspondence is also measured by how parsimoniously the theory is presented. Parsimony is reflected in simplicity of form and economy of words. Simplicity of form refers to the uncluttered description of the elements of the theory, and economy of words refers to the succinctness of the description used to present the theory. In reference to theory validation, the idea of semantic integrity encompasses relationships with general knowledge, soundness of form, clarity and consistency of meaning, and simplicity and economy of words.

The questions related to the correspondence criterion are:

1. Does the theory fit with the established general knowledge about Man and health?

2. Does the theory interrelate concepts at the same level of discourse to describe, explain, or predict about Man and health?

3. With what paradigmatic perspective does the theory correspond?

4. Does the theory correspond with the philosophical assumptions?

5. Are the principles, concepts, and propositions described parsimoniously in abstract terms?

6. Is the meaning of the principles, concepts, and propositions clear?

7. Is the meaning of each concept of the theory at a consistent level of discourse?

Coherence

The coherence criterion is inherent in correspondence but more specifically refers to the syntax of the theory, the internal logic and consistency in the flow of ideas, and the relationship of the theory to others (Kaplan, 1964). Syntax is related to the logical precision with which the ideas of the theory are presented. Logical precision is evident in the organization and movement of the central ideas of the theory from the philosophical assumptions to the propositions. Organization and movement are demonstrated through symmetry and beauty. Symmetry refers to the balance and harmony in the descriptions of the various concepts. The harmony is revealed in the logical congruence of the propositions with the philosophical assumptions. Beauty is the aesthetic way the theory is set forth. Augros and Stanciu (1984) specified that beauty is a primary standard of truth; it is inherent in the combination of logical precision, clarity, and harmony. Beauty also refers to appearance and pleasantness to the eye (Kaplan, 1964).

In reference to theory validation, coherence refers to logical precision, balance, and attractiveness. The specific questions related to the coherence criterion are:

1. How do the principles of the theory relate to other theories?

2. Is there a logical flow from philosophical assumptions to propositions?

3. Is the theory structured in a symmetrically aesthetic way?

Pragmatics

Pragmatics is the theory validation criterion that refers to the function of the theory. The function of a theory is evaluated by evidence that it can be useful in guiding research and practice. This criterion is met if propositions stated at a lower level of abstraction can be derived from the theory and if they can serve as guides to practice and be tested in research. The pragmatics criterion also includes an evaluation of the overall contribution of the theory to nursing science. In reference to theory validation, pragmatics refers to the theory's usefulness as a guide to research and practice and its contribution to nursing science.

The questions related to the pragmatics criterion are:

1. Can the theory be moved down the ladder of abstraction for use in research and practice?

2. Does the theory generate research questions for investigation?

3. Does the theory offer guidelines for practice?

4. Is there evidence in research and practice of support for the theory?

5. How can the contribution of the theory to nursing science be described?

Nurse scholars have set forth frameworks and specified theories from the totality and simultaneity paradigms over the past two decades. Research guided by these frameworks and theories is in process and is being published in the scientific journals of the discipline. Doctoral programs are continuing to prepare researchers for the scientific tasks ahead. The present activity in theory development and research portends a viable future with further expansion and specification of nursing science.

REFERENCES

Augros, R. M., and Stanciu, G. N. (1984). *The new story of science.* Bluff, IL: Regnery Gateway.

Chinn, P. L., and Jacobs, M. K. (1983). *Theory and nursing: A systematic approach.* St. Louis: C. V. Mosby Co.

Duffey, M., and Muhlenkamp, A. F. (1974). A framework for theory analysis, *Nursing Outlook, 22* (9):570-574.

Ellis, R. (1968). Characteristics of significant theories. *Nursing Research, 17* (3): 217-222.

Fawcett, J. (1984). *Analysis and evaluation of conceptual models.* Philadelphia: F. A. Davis Co.

Fitzpatrick, J., and Whall, A. (1983). *Conceptual models of nursing: Analysis and application.* Bowie, MD: Brady Communications.

Hall, L. E. (1966). Another view of nursing care and quality. *In* K. M. Straub and K. S. Parker, eds, *Continuity of patient care: The role of nursing.* Washington, DC: Catholic University Press, pp. 47-60.

Hardy, M. E. (1974). Theories: Components, development, evaluation. *Nursing Research*, 23(2):100-107.

Henderson, V. (1955) *The nature of nursing*. Reprinted in M. E. Meyers, ed, *Nursing fundamentals*. Dubuque, IA: William C. Brown Co.

Johnson, D. E. (1980). The behavioral system for nursing. *In* J. P. Riehl and C. Roy, eds, *Conceptual models for nursing practice*. 2nd ed. New York: Appleton-Century-Crofts, pp. 207-216.

Kaplan, A. (1964). *The conduct of inquiry*. Scranton: Chandler Publishing Co.

Kim, H. S. (1983). *The nature of theoretical thinking in nursing*. New York: Appleton-Century-Crofts.

King, I. M. (1981). *A theory for nursing: Systems, concepts, process*. New York: John Wiley & Sons.

Kuhn, T. S. (1970). *The structure of scientific revolutions*. Chicago: Chicago University Press.

Levine, M. E. (1973). *Introduction to clinical nursing*. 2nd ed. Philadelphia: F. A. Davis Co.

Meleis, A. I. (1985). *Theoretical nursing: Development and progress*. Philadelphia: J. B. Lippincott Co.

Nightingale, F. (1969). *Notes on nursing: What it is and what it is not*. New York: Dover Publications. (Unabridged republication of the first American edition, as published in 1860 by D. Appleton & Company.)

Orem, D. E. (1985). *Nursing: Concepts of practice*. New York: McGraw-Hill Book Co.

Orlando, I. J. (1961). *The dynamic nurse-patient relationship: Function, process, and principles*. New York: G. P. Putnam's Sons.

Parse, R. R. (1981). *Man-living-health: A theory of nursing*. New York: John Wiley & Sons.

Parse, R. R., Coyne, A. B., and Smith, M. J. (1985). *Nursing research: Qualitative methods*. Bowie, MD: Brady Communications.

Peplau, H. E. (1952). *Interpersonal relations in nursing*. New York: G. P. Putnam's Sons.

Rogers, M. E. (1970). *An introduction to the theoretical basis of nursing*. Philadelphia, F. A. Davis.

Rogers, M. E. (1980). Nursing: A science of unitary man. *In* J. P. Riehl and C. Roy, eds, *Conceptual models for nursing practice*. 2nd ed. New York: Appleton-Century-Crofts, pp. 329-337.

Roy, C. (1976). *Introduction to Nursing: An Adaptation Model*. Englewood Cliffs, NJ: Prentice-Hall.

Roy, C. (1984). *Introduction to nursing: An adaptation model*. 2nd ed. Englewood Cliffs, NJ: Prentice-Hall.

Roy, C., and Roberts, S. (1981). *Theory construction in nursing: An adaptation model*. Englewood Cliffs, NJ: Prentice-Hall.

Stevens, B. J. (1984). *Nursing theory*. Boston: Little, Brown & Co.

Walker, L. O., and Avant, K. C. (1983). *Strategies for theory construction in nursing*. New York: Appleton-Century-Crofts.

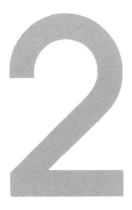

Nursing Science: A Historical Perspective

HILDEGARD E. PEPLAU

In 1974 Armiger said, "There exists today an unprecedented need for identification of the uniqueness of nursing science and practice, lest overriding forces in contemporary society lead to disintegration of nursing as a distinct profession" (pp. 160–164). The phrase, "uniqueness of nursing science and practice," a recurrent refrain in nursing circles, is debatable but the warning still applies. There are characteristics common to all sciences and professions, with the exception of the phenomena central to each field, that are diagnosed, treated, and researched. Nevertheless, there is some urgency in the matter of nursing science in understanding what it is and in developing it more fully and more rapidly in the foreseeable future.

The title of this chapter implies that a nursing science has already emerged, that its emergence can be traced historically, and

13

that evidence in support of the claim can be supplied. Indeed, what distinguishes the history of nursing in the last three decades, and sets that period apart from what went before, is the birth of nursing science. At this juncture no one can foretell all of the changes nursing will undergo in the decades and centuries ahead.

There are many good reasons for the profession to declare the reality of nursing science, granting that its full development has not yet been realized; indeed, no science is ever at its ultimate boundary. Still, nursing science is but a fledgling. It is of interest that, in terms of the contextual nature of science (its social basis) nursing science has become visible in this 20th century, "the century of science." Nursing as a function of women is surely as old as time; nursing as an organized profession having schools in which to educate novices is barely more than a century old in this country. If the beginnings of nursing science are sought in relation to the nursing function, its development has been exceedingly slow; if the starting point is placed in American schools of nursing, a short 111 years ago, then nursing science has progressed rather rapidly.

Nursing has been and still is largely a women's profession. Social circumstances—even in this century, as in times past—have impinged on and erected barriers to nursing's development. The profession's advancement as a science awaited the full development of opportunities for women to learn, and to use their intelligence, particularly to engage in rigorous, disciplined, complex, scientific work. Nurses have slowly but surely surmounted those barriers and have established the beginnings of a nursing science. Nurses are moving steadily forward in terms of their social commitment to improve nursing services, the main purpose of nursing science.

Nursing as a profession—a defined field having authority for its work, codified in laws such as the nursing practice acts—has a social right and a public obligation to develop nursing science. The nurse practice acts generated by state legislators represent the will of the people and therefore imply a reciprocal social contract. That contract obligates nursing not only to provide services, but also to improve them through research and to alter them in light of both changing social need and the findings of research, toward promoting the public's health. Society, on the other hand, has an obligation to provide the essential resources the profession requires for accomplishing its entire mission. Resources in support of the development of nursing science, both private and public, have never been sufficient in terms of the size of the task; nor have research funds been readily forthcoming. Viewed from these perspectives, the emergence and the progress of nursing science to date have been remarkable.

Nursing science has its deepest roots in modern science, which had its birth in the Renaissance between the 15th and 18th centuries, but its flowering surfaced only in the aftermath and continues into current time. It was in these earlier centuries that the three male-dominated professions—theology, law, and medicine—were spawned out of a religious matrix, as was the vocation of nursing. Among the many issues of the earlier days was the question of who "owned" healing, which was a covert activity of women, and therefore of "nurses." Healing was believed to occur by "the will of God," and thus required the intervention of the clergy to intercede for purposes of healing. Meanwhile, women and the "nurses" among them, employed folk methods, common sense, and word-of-mouth transmission of information on what worked to promote healing. In the long run, both theology and nursing lost the healing function to medicine, and for the same reasons—they did not experiment and seek scientific explanations for what was effective in their work, and they did not publish what they learned about illness phenomena, healing functions, and methods.

One of the major institutions in which science is a central feature is the university, the "Empire of the Learned" (Boorstin, 1983). Women and nurses have only relatively recently, and with great difficulty, been accepted into these bastions of learning and sciences. By the 15th century, books were more available than previously, and medical education had already moved into the university. The prevailing language was Latin; women were not taught Latin.

Nursing was a hands-on vocation, and "gentlemen" who studied in university were not to "use their hands"—it was not in keeping with being "learned" (Fraser, 1966). Despite the wealthy women and Mothers Superior who established and ran the early hospitals and asylums, with women volunteers, until nursing became a gainful occupation during the Industrial Revolution, "nurses" were disqualified for university study. The language obstacle, the nature of the work of "nurses," and conceptions about "women's place" in the scheme of things were among the obstacles to academic education in earlier days.

The struggle in the United States to establish nursing schools within academia was not exactly easy, nor is it yet entirely over. At the turn of the century, and well into the 1940s, student nurses in training schools established by hospitals rather than by nurses were taught almost entirely by physicians. Now, it is a well-known principle that the one who teaches controls the content of an occupation. Thus, a supply of nurse teachers was of the utmost priority for the eventual control of the profession by nurses. In 1907, a Department of Nursing was established at Teachers College of Columbia University to provide an opportunity for the academic preparation of teachers of nursing. Baccalaureate programs in nursing were begun in 1893 at Howard University and in 1909 at the University of Minnesota and provided the pool of students for graduate study. It is estimated that by 1936 66 colleges and universities had baccalaureate programs.

Graduate programs in nursing began in the 1940s and had their greatest growth after World War II and into the 1970s. During that quarter century period, one of optimism and generosity, foundation and government funds became available for the support of academic-based nursing education. The eventual visibility of nursing science rested on these developments. In the 1960s, government funds in support of nursing research enabled the preparation of "nurse scientists." Faculty research development grants (21 programs between 1958 and 1966) and various other research projects were launched. It can be argued that, with these developments, nursing in this country had achieved more than a toe-hold in the "Empire of Learning."

Traditions, habits, and patterns of thinking, however, are exceedingly resistant to change. It was not easy for registered nurse students and their hospital-trained teachers, in early baccalaureate programs, to shift away from the subservience, and docility that all too many nurses had obediently acquired as nurse attitudes. Many were not attuned, and some not sympathetic, to university traditions of research and scholarship. The contemplative, reflective mode, requiring analysis, critique, and thought about one's field, which is characteristic of the university at its best, seemed to some antithetical to nursing's activity orientation, to the "learning by doing." In the 1930s and 1940s a number of studies were implemented to determine the functions of nurses. The question then was what did nurses do, not what did they know. Similarly, nurse practice acts specified functions and mostly defined nursing as "the art and science of nursing." The question "what is the focus for nursing research?" has been asked only within the past two to three decades. It arose simultaneously with the more embarrassing one, "what is nursing?" Undaunted, nurses searched for and found answers for both of these questions—not answers for all time, but for now, for current uses in the advancement of nursing as a profession.

Thinking about nursing as a separate profession, different from and only at times complementary to medicine, was to many nurses a new idea. Yet if there was such an endeavor as nursing research, surely nursing had to be differentiated from medicine and the work of nurses had to be separated out from prevailing all-encompassing views of medical care. The phenomenon of concern, the domain of the nursing profession, had to be identified, for the territory is germane to the research. Among other purposes, nursing science, and all other sciences, aim to explain phenomena it seeks to control as its socially delegated responsibility. There are many modes of explanation of phenomena—intuition, common sense, received beliefs from authority figures, rule of thumb—all common in earlier days in nursing, and all having to be superceded by scientific thinking, disciplined thought, and systematic inquiry. The nurses' perceptions of their work, their place, and their responsibility as women in academia had to be rethought, reshaped, and reoriented toward a new conception of nursing, a new kind of social institution in which it was taught, and ultimately toward evolving a new conception of nursing science.

While looking forward, the nursing profession, often glances back to the founder of modern nursing, who, in today's parlance was more a role model than a promoter of nursing science. Florence Nightingale was a scientist, no doubt the first nurse who merits that appellation. Covel (in Levin, 1980), says this about her:

Over the centuries, society's interest in the quality of health care has been surprisingly muted. While references to concern about quality can be traced to Hippocrates, the first recorded analytical approach was Florence Nightingale's effort to develop a reporting system to provide patient care data, profiles, and outcomes (expressed as mortality rates) in an attempt to improve the care provided to casualties of the Crimean War. Her agenda reads very much like the one being proposed for the 1980's. (p. 113)

Boorstin (1983) has pointed out that Nightingale was "the unlikely champion" of the then-new science of statistics, and promoted it as one of her "proclaimed religious duties." A well-marked copy of *Social Physics*, a book by Adolphe Quetelet (1796-1874), who enlarged the term statistics to include "data about mankind," was found among Nightingale's (1820-1910) possessions when she died. Measurement of phenomena is considered a criteria of modern day science; Nightingale was surely one of its earliest and able practitioners. Whether she encouraged and educated other nurses for scientific research or recognized that "nursing science is the source to make explicit, sound conceptual frameworks for the practice of nursing" (Donaldson and Crowley, 1978, p. 118) is a question for a historian and is beyond the scope of this paper. What is likely, however, is that Nightingale was exposed to preconceptions about women, associated with Victorian England and with the Industrial Revolution, particularly as these were played out in England during her formative years.

In the 19th century and in centuries before that, it was considered acceptable for a few upper-class women, such as Nightingale, to use their intelligence—to think—providing such a woman was unmarried and childless. In that event, however, such a woman was more or less tolerated as an aberration who "thought like a man." Of course, up to (if not into) the mid-20th century, student nurses were discouraged from marriage and in some schools also from thinking. Well into the 1940s, many textbooks for nurses, often written by physicians, clergy, or psychologists, reminded nurses that theory was too much for them, that nurses did not need to think but rather merely to follow rules, be obedient, be compassionate, do their "duty," and carry out medical orders. Despite such admonitions, the history of nursing shows that there were quite a few nurses who thought very seriously about their profession, plotted the direction of its future, and steered it toward academic-based nursing education and nursing research.

Parsons (1968) wrote that science is first and foremost an intellectual discipline. Gortner and Nahm (1977), in an informative paper entitled "An Overview of Nursing Research in the United States," provided ample examples that "intellectual discipline" has been in evidence since schools of nursing were established in this country in 1873. At the turn of the century and up to its midpoint, there were many important research studies. Furthermore, nurses were speaking out about a wide variety of health problems, publishing scholarly papers and case studies, and addressing issues of the profession in a forceful manner. However, while citing these noteworthy intellectual efforts, Gortner and Nahm stated that, "During the past 30 years nursing research has come into its own. Ever-increasing numbers of nurses are involved in nursing research and in preparation of nurses to do research" (1977, p. 10). This finding, which results from a substantive survey of nursing literature, supports the recent emergence of both a stronger trend of "intellectual discipline" and of "nursing science."

One significant criterion applied to determine whether a field can be designated as a science is the availability of a group of educated researchers intimately knowledgeable about that field. With great care, Gortner and Nahm (1977) have documented in detail the research resources and other evidence that show that nursing science meets this criterion.

Philosophers of science point out that there are two ways by which scientific knowledge in a particular field is achieved: (1) theoretical knowledge accumulates, by accretion, extant theories being revised by new scientific findings from research; and (2) new and revised knowledge, especially profound discoveries, result from shifts from one paradigm to another. Popper (1968), for example, wrote that:

. . . *Science should be visualized as progressing* from problems—to problems of ever-increasing depth. For a scientific theory—an exploratory theory—is, if anything, an attempt to solve a scientific problem, that is to say, a problem concerned or connected with the discovery of an explanation . . . our theories may precede, historically, even our problems. *Yet* science starts only with problems (p. 222).

Kuhn (1970), while in agreement about cumulative knowledge, which he called "normal science," proposed that sciences advance more significantly, dramatically, as a consequence of a shift in paradigms that guide the activity of a given scientific community (p. 10).

A paradigm is an overriding idea that markedly changes the ways of looking at a field's phenomena. ("the world is flat" vs. "the world is round"). It is a model "from which spring[s] particular coherent traditions of scientific research," which serves "for a time implicitly to define the legitimate problems and methods of a research field for succeeding generations of practitioners" (p. 10). There are two essential characteristics of a paradigm. First, the achievement is sufficiently unprecedented to attract an enduring group away from competing modes of activity, and second, it is sufficiently open-ended to leave all sorts of problems for the redefined group of practitioners to resolve (p. 10). Kuhn also claimed that paradigms characterize "mature science" and that a change in paradigm can be called a revolution"; at least they seem so to the affected adherents, to others they may "seem normal parts of the developmental process" (pp. 92–93). The issue of "normal science" vs. "paradigm" is an *and/but* one rather that an *either/or* controversy.

The issue is relevant to this chapter. An important publication by Brown and others (1984), entitled "Nursing's Search for Scientific Knowledge," focuses on efforts toward "a cumulative science" and merely mentions in passing the matter of paradigms. This article, like the Gortner-Nahm one, also cites 1952 as "a turning point"; the launching of the journal *Nursing Research* confirmed "the profession's commitment to scholarship and science. . . ." The publication documented these facts: (1) that the amount of nursing research has increased; (2) that it has become more clinically focused; (3) that it has demonstrated a greater theoretical orientation; and (4) that it has shown greater sophistication in research methods. Concluded the authors, "However, the major limitation of the nursing research reviewed was judged to be its non-cumulative nature," a similar point having been made by at least four other authors in the 1977–1980 period cited in the Brown work.

In the past decade, if not somewhat earlier, there has been unprecedented, almost "feverish," activity in relation to nursing theory, particularly in academic-based schools of nursing. Faculty and students are discussing the nature of the work of this or that "nurse theorist," and books comparing nursing's many theoretical models are already available, in press, or being written. It may be that all of this critique and intellectual activity regarding "nursing theories" portends the eventual demise or synthesis of some of them into "normal science," that is, background knowledge or the supremacy of one model to guide nursing research in the years ahead.

There are at present different, competing models in nursing. Fawcett (1984) has examined seven of them: Johnson's behavioral system, King's open systems, Levine's conservation principles, Neuman's systems, Orem's self-care, Roger's life process, and Roy's adaptation. The list omits the works of Norris (1964), Parse (1981), and Peplau (1952), and no doubt others. Nursing is surely moving away from its "empirical, rule-of-thumb" practice toward being a theory-oriented professional practice.

Based on a review of nursing literature, Donaldson and Crowley (1978) have formulated "three general themes for inquiry" that in their judgment show "remarkable consistency in the recurrent themes that nurse scholars use to explain what they conceive to be the essence or core of nursing" (p. 113). This framework is in the direction of a synthesis of the works of many nurse scholars and includes some aspects of the models previously mentioned.

As early as 1964, Norris, a nurse theorist, published a paper in which overall concept of health and illness were presented in order to pursue a research method by which the "unique content" of a nursing science could be obtained. The framework was then used to explore the phenomenon of "bedtime as a therapeutic regime" (Norris, 1964). Norris's model proposed not only a method for analyzing a phenomenon, but it also showed its relation to the larger core, health and illness, from which it was derived, and it laid out the relations among parts of the example of the model that required systematic study in order to achieve explanatory theory. It showed the enormous complexity of nursing science.

Fawcett (1984) has proposed "the metaparadigm of nursing," which was constructed by using four concepts drawn from literature and the three themes from the Donaldson and Crowley paper, and which showed research already completed and derived from the seven models discussed in her book. Whether this effort reflects a bent within the profession for cohesion, or suggests a unified field theory of nursing, and, therefore, a lack of distinct, different, self-contained knowledge in the paradigms thus merged, merits critique and debate. One thing is certain: for the first time in nursing's history, there are competing paradigms of nursing, each having a group of adherents—nurse scholars and scientists—seeking to use one or the other paradigm to clarify if not influence the field of nursing and nursing research. There ought to be intense conflict, argument, discussion, and comparisons of performance in research to challenge each of these paradigms. That would be a healthy sign showing that intellectual vigor and rigor are alive in nursing.

At least one other document ought to be mentioned. It is the 1980 publication of the American Nursing Association (ANA), *Nursing: A Social Policy Statement*. The ANA's definition of nursing constitutes a shift away from all other previous definitions (ANA, 1980). It provides "defining characteristics of nursing practice" in relation to the nursing process and standards of practice (ANA, 1980, pp. 14-15). It was drawn from the New York State Practice Act of 1971 and from similar acts in many states. Unlike all previous definitions of nursing, this one particularly specifies the phenomena of focus in nursing practice, which is at once the core for which explanatory theory derived from nursing research is needed to explain the phenomena, to guide practice, and to provide the conceptual base for nursing education. This document has the additional merit of a growing consensus, among nurses and the public, as its definition of nursing or ones very similar, are already contained in many nursing practice acts. Popularity, of course, is not a criterion that determines that a field is a science; specification of the phenomena of focus, however, is one important criterion by which nursing should be assessed and judged viable as a science. That is what a science is: facts, theories, and a way of knowing and representing phenomena pertaining to a scientific field and the world in which it lives.

Thus far, three criteria by which to judge that a field is a science have been discussed: (1) Science is an intellectual discipline; it requires educated researchers knowledgeable about the particular field of scientific endeavor. (2) The field has some cumulative background knowledge, "normal science," and competing paradigms that provide direction to the research. (3) The phenomenological focus of the field is specified, or foci are inherent or implied in the paradigms. Nursing science meets these criteria; there are others. The phenomena central to a particular field constitute its domain; in the case of professions, it is the area of socially ascribed authority and responsibility; in terms of a science, the domain is the central target of research. Domains shrink by absorption into other professions or sciences and expand by accretion of claims to new phenomena attributable to social change or to new scientific discoveries. The scientific search is for regularities and relations within, across, and among phenomena. In this process it is characteristic of all sciences to order accumulated knowledge through systems of classification. Such taxonomies name or identify the kinds of phenomena, the name providing a common language and clues toward meaning. As knowledge about a field's phenomena accumulates, this classification vocabulary not only catalogues but shows range and variety of units (Boorstin, 1983, p. 424). While all such classification systems are open to revision, there tends to emerge, in time, a constancy, a certain stability to these building blocks. Novices entering a scientific field learn these designations and use them as handles while becoming immersed in the greater complexities of the field of scientific inquiry.

Thus, a *fourth criterion* is an established system of classification of phenomena. Nursing as a profession is in process of developing a nursing diagnosis classification system. Gebbie and Lavin (1975), Gordon (1982), and others, generally called the St. Louis Group, have been at work on such a taxonomy since 1973. One question is whether there is or should be considerable convergence between the phenomena of nursing science endeavors and the developing nursing diagnostic system.

Scientific research has long been considered to be best when it uses instruments, such as statistics, for measurement and for discovery. Brown and others (1984) noted that "since 1970, about as many nursing researchers have employed previously published tools as attempted to originate their own" (p. 30). While there were questions concerning application of instruments, the range and variety was not specified. Measurement, the *fifth criterion of a science,* is one that is being met by nursing.

Merton (1968) framed common characteristics of science, such as those already discussed, in a somewhat different way and added a *sixth criterion* worth considering: "a set of cultural values and mores governing the activities termed scientific" (p. 605). He presents four values that are common traditions in existing sciences: universalism, communism, disinterestedness, and organized skepticism. No study was located that investigated the extent to which these values pervade the nursing community in general and the scientific community of nurse researchers in particular.

Universalism means that ". . . truth claims, whatever their course, are to be subjected to *preestablished impersonal criteria:* consonant with observation and with previously confirmed knowledge" (Merton, 1968, p. 605). In other words, "ethnocentric particularism" is to be avoided. In reviewing a "meticulously documented book" by Rossiter (1982), Lankford (1984) wrote that it "raises serious questions about the role of universalism in American science. It has long been supposed that the norm of universalism will guarantee that scientists are judged on the basis of performance, the papers and books they publish, rather than by irrelevant criteria such as gender or race" (p. 193). Rossiter's (1982) book documents that gender adversely influenced the place of women scientists in universities, and despite the high quality of their scientific work rendered them "invisible." Nurse researchers, at least those of more than a decade ago, surely have known the principle of universalism intellectually and on occasion its opposite experientially.

Communism as Merton (1968) uses the term refers to "common ownership": "The substantive findings of science are a product of social collaboration and are assigned to the community. They constitute a common heritage in which the equity of the individual producer is severly limited" (p. 605). In other words, the rewards for discovery of a theory are "recognition and esteem" and not ownership. The contributions of nursing science to the larger scientific community have not yet been extensive enough to raise issues related to this value; nursing has, however, open access to any published theory for application in nursing practice or in nursing research. This principle, if applied, lays to rest the question of "uniqueness of nursing science."

Merton wrote that disinterestedness is "not to be equated with altruism nor interested action with egoism. . . . It is rather a distinctive pattern of institutional control of a wide range of motives which characterize the behavior of scientists" (1968, p. 609). The nursing profession is very high on altruism and philosophy. Indeed, there seems to be an extensive nursing ideology, a long tradition of concern, caring, and interestedness, the opposite of this norm of science.

Organized skepticism "is both a methodologic and institutional mandate. The suspension of judgment until 'the facts are at hand' and the detached scrutiny of beliefs in terms of empirical and logical criteria. . . ." (Merton, 1968, p. 614). Gortner and Nahm (1977, p. 26) have stated that the purpose of the first ANA nursing research conference in 1964 was "to provide opportunity for nurses engaged in research to examine critically . . ." the work presented. "The objective of critical examination was taken as a mandate . . . and its literal interpretation by participants and presenters created some awkward moments" (p. 26). That comment states diplomatically that some presenters were quite upset by critiques of their work. Nurses then were very much oriented to getting approval, being liked, and all too often viewed a critique of work as personal disapproval. The ability to tolerate skepticism among nurses, and particularly among nurse researchers, has developed and is evidenced in the many research conferences now held annually across the country. In any case, the scientific community of nurses ought to be encouraged toward vigorous skepticism and even noisy debate.

Of the six criteria presented and discussed briefly, by which a judgment can be made that nursing science is a viable reality as claimed, nursing easily meets five of them and most probably the sixth one, on values, as well.

Public recognition of the products of science is both confirmation of its existence and one very useful route for increasing public and private support of research. The public's imagination is more readily captured when the reported research findings are connected to the daily life concerns of citizens. A case in point is Eland (1984, p. 38), who, "as a nurse and research scientist had dedicated herself to children in pain. For ten years, she worked to develop a technique called the Eland Color Tool, which helps determine the precise location and amount of pain that children experience in everything from severe burn injuries and cancer to routine dental work." Using this assessment tool, Eland is now working on pain reduction methods.

The instance presented also raises the question as to whether nursing science is basic, applied, or both. So-called "pure" or basic science characteristically pursues investigation or experiment for the sake of knowledge with no obvious or immediate practical use envisioned as a consequence of the research. That there may be or are payoffs in the long run is beside the point. Applied science, on the other hand, involves research aimed from the onset toward a practical outcome. It would be tragic for the scientific community of nurses to see the pure vs. applied controversy as an either/or proposition. Surely all nurse researchers, scientists, and scholars should follow their own inclinations in this matter. Medwar (in Judson, 1980, p. 3) said that "great science is conceived at the boundary where exact observation confronts leaping imagination," and further, that "you must feel in yourself an exploratory impulsion—an acute discomfort at incomprehension—and relieve that through searching to know" (p. 5). The form of the search, pure or applied, ought to be dictated by the incomprehended phenomenon or problem and by the competence of the research scientist, and not by an a priori decision by the profession. Nursing science can be both pure and applied.

It is, however, a fact that an immediate need of the profession is for a scientifically derived theoretical underpinning for the practice of nursing, as Lindeman (1985) has urged. This urgency, however, ought not to preclude nurse researchers from searching in other directions.

One of the questions not yet discussed in this chapter is who first used the phrase "nursing science" and under what circumstances. In 1963, Rogers edited a new journal entitled *Nursing Science*, and Peplau (1952, p. 261) had used the phrase in 1952. To continue the search before that time would be difficult; actually, the fact may not be relevant. After all, the term statistics was first used in 1672 but it was more than a century later that Quetelt was designated the founder of this field on the basis of more substantial work than using a word (Boorstin, 1983, p. 672). Early medicine had its "Aristolelians," "Galenists," and "Paracelsians" and contemporary nursing has its Royers, Kingians, Rogerians, Oremsians, Parseons, and others—all explorers on the frontiers of nursing science.

The journal *Isis* publishes articles on the history of science. Nursing science is not mentioned in this journal. Rossiter's survey and book documenting the struggles of women scientists in this country up to 1940, also does not mention nursing. But then it wasn't until 1946 that the U.S. Bureau of the Census classified nurses as professionals rather than as domestics. A recent paper (Garling and others, 1985) published in *Nursing Outlook*, comparing the impact of the Flexner (1910 medicine) and the Goldmark (1923 nursing) Reports, conveys not only the facts but the climate of opinion within medicine, nursing, and the public regarding these two professions and their educational requirements. The whole history of relationships between men and women, from the 12th to the 20th centuries, is reflected in the differential treatment of these two reports.

At this point, nursing has achieved much: it meets the criteria of a science; it has an honorary society, Sigma Theta Tau, composed of the best and brightest; it has the American Academy of Nursing, of which intellectual leaders are members; and it has the ANA Council of Nurse Researchers. There are countless research conferences for nurses annually and have been since 1964. Nurses have been elected to membership in the National Academy of Sciences since 1970. There are nursing research journals. The list could go on; yet the work that lies ahead is enormous in scope.

This is not the time for nurses to sit on their profession's laurels. For a quarter century (1945–1971), the nursing profession in this country moved ahead swiftly and significantly, using every opportunity and federal dollar of support that was available. Now there are countervailing forces, conservatism, retrenchment, cost-containment, a post-industrial era producing social changes and ambiguity, an oversupply of physicians and other trends, and maybe even a backlash for the progress so recently achieved by the nursing profession. If there ever was a time when the products of nursing science were needed, it is now and in the coming decade. For, as we approach the 21st century, we have all the components of a nursing science that is just beginning to guide the nursing profession into an ever-more useful future for its services to people.

REFERENCES

American Nurses Association (1980). *Nursing: A social policy statement.* Kansas City, MO: ANA.

Armiger, B. (1974). Scholarship in nursing. *Nursing Outlook, 22*:160-164.

Boorstin, D. J. (1983). *The discoverers: A history of man's search to know his world and himself.* New York: Random House, pp. 424, 489, 672, 674.

Brown, J. S., Tanner, C. A., and Padrick, K. P. (1984). Nursing's search for scientific knowledge. *Nursing Research, 33*(1):26-32.

Donaldson, S. K., and Crowley, D. M. (1978). The discipline of nursing. *Nursing Outlook, 26*(2):113-118.

Eland, J. (1984). The best of the new generation: Men and women under forty who are changing America. *Esquire*, December, p. 38.

Fawcett, J. (1984). *Analysis and evaluation of conceptual models of nursing.* Philadelphia: F. A. Davis Co.

Fawcett, J. (1984). The metaparadigm of nursing: Present status and future refinements. *Image, 16*(3):84-87.

Fraser, A. (1966). *The weaker vessel.* New York: Alfred A. Knopf, p. 544.

Garling, J. (1985). Flexner and Goldmark: Why the difference in impact. *Nursing Outlook, 33*(1):26-31.

Gebbie, K. M., and Lavin, M. A., eds. (1975). *Classification of nursing diagnosis*, Proceedings of First National Conference. St. Louis: C. V. Mosby.

Gordon, M. (1982). *Manual of nursing diagnosis.* New York: McGraw-Hill Book Co.

Gortner, S. R., and Nahm, H. (1977). An overview of nursing research in the United States. *Nursing Research, 26*(1):10-28.

Judson, H. F. (1980). *The search for solutions.* New York: Holt, Rinehart & Winston, pp. 3, 5.

Kuhn, T. S. (1970). *The structure of scientific revolutions.* Chicago: Chicago University Press.

Lankford, J. (1984). Book review, Review Symposia. *Isis, 75* (1):276.

Levin, A., ed. (1980). *Regulating health care: The struggle for control.* New York: New York Academy of Political Science, p. 113.

Lindeman, C. (1985). Theory and research as basic to nursing practice. *Am. Nurse*, Feb., p. 19.

Merton, R. K. (1968). *Social theory and social structure.* New York: Free Press, pp. 605-614.

Norris, C. M. (1964). Toward a science of nursing. *Nursing Forum, 3* (3):10-45.

Nursing Science (1963). Philadelphia: F. A. Davis Co.

Parse, R. R. (1981). *Man-living-health: A theory of nursing.* New York: John Wiley & Sons.

Parsons, T. (1968). Professions. *In International encyclopedia of the social sciences*, vol. 12. New York: Macmillan, pp. 536-547.

Peplau, H. E. (1952). *Interpersonal relations in nursing.* New York: G. P. Putnam's Sons.

Popper, K. A. (1968). *Conjectures and refutations: The growth of scientific knowledge*. New York: Harper Torchbooks.
Rossiter, M. W. (1982). *Women scientists in America: Struggles and strategies to 1940*. Baltimore: Johns Hopkins University Press.

Section Overview

THE TOTALITY PARADIGM

ROSEMARIE RIZZO PARSE

The Man-environment totality paradigm is the predominant worldview in nursing today. Historically, this paradigm rooted in one view of the works of Nightingale (1969) has been supported and promoted over time as the discipline of nursing evolved. It is a natural outgrowth of nursing's close connection with medicine, focusing heavily on the natural science view of Man as the total sum of parts. As a paradigm gives rise to theories that guide practice and research, it has been the totality paradigm that has created the major impact to date on nursing research and practice.

The totality paradigm differs from the simultaneity paradigm in three significant ways: in the assumptions about Man and health, in the goals of nursing, and in the implications for research and practice.

Assumptions About Man and Health

In the totality paradigm, Man is considered a bio-psycho-socio-spiritual organism whose environment can be manipulated to maintain or promote balance. Man interacts with the environment, establishes transactions, and plans toward goal attainment. Capable of self-care, Man is an adapting organism who may require assistance with coping and meeting some self-care demands. Health is viewed in this paradigm as being a dynamic state and process of physical, psychological, social, and spiritual well-being (Parse and others, 1985). It is something Man has, which can be made better by manipulation of the environment. There is an optimal level of health toward which Man strives. The theoretical roots related to a totality view of Man are broadly grounded in the works of Helson (1964), Selye (1946), Sullivan (1953), Maslow (1970), Newton (1934), and Descartes (1960). The language of the theories in this paradigm is specified at a level that is readily connected with the traditional practice of nursing. While the conceptualizations in the theories are systematized in structures useful for nursing, the ideas are closely associated with medical science.

Goals of Nursing

The goals of nursing in the totality paradigm focus on health promotion, care and cure of the sick, and prevention of illness. Those receiving nursing care are persons designated as ill by societal norms. Frameworks and theories from this paradigm guide practices that focus on helping sick individuals to adapt, care for themselves, and attain health goals. Care during illness, prevention of disease, and maintenance and promotion of health are the important aspects of nursing practice. The authority figure in regard to nursing and the prime decision maker in this paradigm is the nurse. There are systematized nursing care plans for persons with the various health problems identified by medical science, which are modified to meet individual needs. The outcomes of nursing practice can be measured by the level of adaptation, the self-care agency, and the goals attained by persons receiving nursing care.

Implications for Research and Practice

The process of nursing research that tests theories from the totality paradigm is by nature quantitative. The quantitative methods borrowed from the natural sciences are fundamentally consistent with the beliefs about Man in this paradigm in that they test causal and associative relationships. Use of these methods is appropriate while nursing science is developing, but research methods evolving directly from the theories of the discipline are required in all sciences.

Nursing practice based on totality paradigm theories is made operational through the traditional nursing process of assessing, diagnosing, planning, implementing, and evaluating. This is not a practice methodology grounded in the paradigm, but rather the problem-solving process elaborated upon for nursing. Nursing science requires unique practice methodologies in the totality paradigm that focus on the processes involved in helping a person adapt to illness, become more capable of self-care, and set realistic goals.

Roy (1984), Orem (1985), and King (1981) creatively synthesized systematized structures consistent with the beliefs about Man and health in the totality paradigm to guide research and practice. The following chapters consist of original works by these theorists.

who describe the essences of their theories. A critique
of the theory, using the criteria set forth in Chapter
One, follows each chapter.

REFERENCES

Descartes, R. (1960). *A discourse on method and meditations*, trans. by L. J.
    LaFleur. New York: Liberal Arts Press.
Helson, H. (1964). *Adaptation level theory*. New York: Harper & Row.
King, I. M. (1981). *A theory for nursing*. New York: John Wiley & Sons.
Maslow, A. (1970). *Motivation and personality*, 2nd ed. New York: Harper &
    Row.
Newton, I. (1934). *Mathematical principles of natural philosophy and system of
    the world*, trans. by A. Mott. Berkeley, CA: University of California Press.
Nightingale, F. (1969). *Notes on nursing: What it is and what it is not.* New York,
    Dover Publications. (Unabridged republication of the first American edition,
    as published in 1860 by D. Appleton & Company.)
Orem, D. E. (1985). *Nursing concepts of practice.* New York: McGraw-Hill.
Roy, C. (1984). *Introduction to nursing: An adaptation model.* Englewood Cliffs,
    NJ: Prentice-Hall.
Selye, H. (1946). The general adaptation syndrome and diseases of adaptation.
    *Journal of Allergy, 17:*231, 289, 358.
Sullivan, H. S. (1953). *The interpersonal theory of psychiatry.* New York:
    W. W. Norton and Co.

3

Roy's Adaptation Model

CALLISTA ROY

EDITORIAL PERSPECTIVE

Roy (1984) has characterized Man an organism with cognator and regulator systems and four modes of adaptation: physiologic, self-concept, role function, and interdependence. This language describes Man consistent with the totality paradigm. The modes closely follow the view of Man as a particulate being. The notion of environment for Roy (1984) is that it consists of focal, contextual, and residual stimuli, and that it can be manipulated to promote adaptation and maintain health. Roy has defined health as both a state and a process, a definition that is also consistent with the totality paradigm view.

Her idea of health as a process is a new addition to Roy's (1984) definition of health, and though it appears her thinking was influenced by some newer views set forth in the simultaneity paradigm, the process of health she refers to is the process of adaptation. This means that Man copes with and adapts to the environment—again, an idea in keeping with the totality paradigm.

In the following chapter, Roy (1984) explains her model of adaptation and elaborates on her beliefs about Man, environment, health, and nursing. She identifies Man's modes of adaptation, the mechanisms for coping, the three environmental stimuli, and discusses research and practice implications related to her model.

Introduction

This chapter conveys the assumptions, concepts, and principles of the Roy Adaptation Model of nursing with a focus on historical development, current views, and future directions, as well as a focus on work accomplished as a clinical nurse scholar in neuroscience nursing.

Nursing knowledge is related to nursing models. Consider the notion used by Donaldson and Crowley (1978), who surveyed nursing literature through the years and focused on commonalities. They identified research that focused on nursing's concern with principles and laws that govern the life processes, well-being and optimal functioning of human beings, whether sick or well, and on nursing's concern with both the pattern of human behavior in interaction with the environment and the processes by which positive changes in health status are affected.

This leads to the firm conviction that nursing knowledge can be focused in two major areas: on the processes by which people positively affect their health status, and on nursing actions to enhance these processes. From this can be derived a definition of nursing science: the developing system of knowledge about persons, which, through its theorizing and research, will observe, classify, and relate those processes by which persons positively affect their health status, and the practice by which nurses enhance these processes.

The nursing model clarifies and articulates a notion of person, environment, health, and nursing. The resulting theories and research lead first to the basic science of nursing (the human life processes), and then to nursing practice (the theories and research related to what nursing does to enhance these processes). In this chapter, definitions of a model and theory are not based on order of generality, even though that notion is reflected in the literature, particularly in Fawcett (1984). Rather, a model can be as abstract or as concrete as desired. The models of the artificial hearts that are being transplanted are very concrete. By the same notion very broad theories of social change, which consider the rise and fall of civilizations, are distinguished by form and function. In other words, theories are what help relate the concepts and then describe, explain, and make predictions about phenomena. Models provide direction about which theories will help describe people and their life processes and describe what nursing can do about them.

Assumptions of the Roy Model

The assumptions of the Roy Adaptation Model are of two kinds: scientific assumptions (systems theory and Helson's adaptation level theory) and philosophical assumptions (Roy, 1976, 1984).

The systems theory assumptions focus primarily on holism, interdependence, control processes, information feedback, and, most importantly, the highly complex nature of living systems. Helson focused on all behavior as adaptive. He believed that this behavior is the function of both the stimulus coming in, how light or dark it is, how hot the room is, and the adaptation level (Roy, 1984). The process of responding positively as well as very actively is also significant from Helson's view (Roy, 1984).

The Roy model also articulates humanistic assumptions, which basically focus on a person's creative power, purposefulness, holism, viewpoint as a value, and the interpersonal process as significant.

Elements of the Model

Conceptual models in nursing address four major elements—person, environment, health, and nursing—and these are the broad concepts of the Roy Adaptation Model.

PERSON

The first element is person. Nursing focuses on the individual level or the family level, or the level of social organizations and community. The Roy Adaptation Model views the person or group as an adaptive system with coping mechanisms manifested by the adaptive modes.

For the individual person, the coping mechanisms are broadly categorized as regulator and cognator whereas the adaptive modes are identified as physiological function, self-concept, role function, and interdependence. A person receives input from both the internal and external environments and processes these inputs by way of the regulator and cognator systems, which themselves manifest activity in the four modes to produce responses.

The coping mechanisms of the person are innate and acquired ways of responding to a changing environment. The regulator is one way of describing how the person responds automatically to many changes in the environment. Humans are extremely complex in how they interact with the changing world; thus, it seems useful to categorize some of this complexity in a meaningful way for nurses. As an example, the regulator receives input from the external environment and from changes in the person's internal state. It then processes the changes through neurochemical endocrine channels to produce the responses. This is the mechanism that makes it possible for a mother to move fast enough to catch her child from running into the path of a moving car. Without conscious thought, she has received the extra adrenaline and made all the necessary neurochemical responses to meet an emergency situation.

Conversely, the cognator uses both conscious and unconscious cognitive and emotive processes. It responds through the complex mechanisms of perceptual information processing, learning, judgement, and emotion. Thus, the anxiety experienced by the mother for the safety of her toddler may lead her to use a problem-solving skill, such as to decide to put a fence around her yard (Roy and Roberts, 1981; Roy, 1984; Andrews and Roy 1986).

Work presently in progress on the regulator and cognator mechanisms includes efforts to describe and study further these processes, both clinically and in research. For example, people are working on the cognitive processes of patient decision-making. The clinical research focuses on patient information processing with patients recovering from head injury. The purpose is to describe what the cognitive recovery looks like, and thereby learn about a key positive life process, and to develop insights into theory development in this area. The relationship between the regulator and the cognator for the Roy nursing model holds the key to holism. The patient as a whole person can be understood by knowing these processes.

Coping mechanisms are manifested by the adaptive modes. Initially, the adaptive modes were viewed as being what the nurse saw in the person. Later they were considered as a classification of the ways of coping that manifest cognator-regulator activity in four categories—physiological, self-concept, role function, and interdependence—developed from 500 samples of patient behavior. In 1970, students, in implementing the Roy model in a curriculum, were asked to collect samples of patient behavior and categorize them. The information reflects what patients were experiencing in all of the clinical areas—pediatrics, obstetrics, medical-surgical, and community health.

Adaptive Modes

Physiological. Recent developments with the modes have focused primarily on reorganization of the physiological and interdependence modes. Through many revisions with input from educators, clinicians, and theory critics, the physiological mode has been reorganized, and can now be used for nursing assessment and the organization of curriculum content. It focuses on five basic needs in a hierarchy (oxygenation, nutrition, elimination, activity and rest, and protection), and on four regulator processes (the senses, fluid and electrolytes, neurological, and endocrine functions).

Self-Concept. The second adaptive mode is self-concept. Defined as the composite of belief and feelings that one holds about one's self at a given time, it is formed by perception, particularly by others' reactions, and by directing one's behavior.

The behaviors that the nurse assesses under the self-concept mode are divided into the physical self and the personal self. The physical self involves sensation and body image; the personal self involves self-consistency, self-ideal, and the moral-ethical self. Self-consistency is that continuity of self over time, even though feelings change based on what is occurring in one's life. The self-ideal is what one expects of self and what one wants to accomplish. The moral-ethical self involves spiritual values, the goodness of personal lives. The influencing factor, then, for anything in a person's self-concept is perception.

Role Function. The third adaptive mode is role function. This implies that not just the person as self is influenced by health and illness, but their roles as well. How one relates to other people is significant. Roles are defined as the behavior of one person relating to another, with each occupying a given position, for example, teacher-student.

The types of roles are primary, secondary, and tertiary. Primary roles are those that are positions related to one's developmental level, such as generative adult female. Secondary roles are those positions such as wage earner, mother, nurse. Tertiary roles are temporary positions that are related to secondary roles, such as being president of the parent-teacher association. The role function assessment focuses on behaviors that demonstrate achievement of the goals of the roles. These behaviors are related to instrumental behaviors and feelings of satisfaction. The nurse assesses how well the roles are lived out and how satisfying they are to the persons involved.

Interdependence. Interdependence is the fourth adaptive mode. The content changes of the interdependence mode have been significant over the last couple of years. This allows interdependence to be distinguished from self-concept and role function.

Interdependence is a way of maintaining integrity that involves the willingness and ability to love, respect, and value others, and to accept and respond to love, respect, and value given by others. In assessing interdependence, the nurse studies behaviors related to the give and take of these ideas and how they are handled in terms of independent behaviors, such as achieving goals, dependence, and affection seeking. What influences interdependence is the presence of significant others, and whether they are available in the support system. People in the support system can love, value, and respect, but not know how to express these feelings, which is also a part of the interactional skills that relate to growth and development.

The present stage of development related to the element of person prompts another look at the interrelatedness of the four modes and the assessment methodologies within the modes, as well as the related nursing interventions. For example, it is important to study the effect of interdependent relationiships on the development of self-concept.

ENVIRONMENT

The second major element is environment. It was, in fact, the first concept developed, and is based on Helson's view of the adaptation level (Roy, 1981). Helson, who thought learning was adaptation, described human behavior as a total process of adaptation (Roy, 1984). A physiological psychologist who began his work with light-dark adaptation, Helson basically said that adaptive responses are a function of the environmental stimulus. He believes that adaptation level is made up of focal stimuli, immediately confronting a person, and contextual stimuli, all of those factors present in the environment. The residual stimuli are all other factors from the past, which may be relevant but which are not determined to be immediately affecting the person. For Helson these residual stimuli are difficult to identify in a situation.

Environment is in fact all of the internal and external conditions, circumstances, and influences surrounding or affecting the development and behavior of persons or groups. It can be categorized as focal, contextual, and residual stimuli. These categories are useful in the assessment process (Roy, 1984).

HEALTH

The third major element of the model is health. Helson's description or definition of adaptation supports the definition of health (Roy, 1984): a process of responding positively to environmental changes. It is this positive response that decreases the responses necessary to cope with the stimuli and that increases sensitivity to other factors.

Based on Helson's early notions, adaptation level, in an attempt to capture the dynamic aspect of adaptation, has been redefined as a constantly changing point. It is a changing point made up of focal, contextual, and residual stimuli that represents one's own standard and the range of stimuli to which one can respond. This refers to the person in the total life context, including goals of life, activity, and creativity. The criteria in adaptation are that a person's own level is such that it leads to the accomplishment of goals of survival, growth, reproduction, and mastery. The adaptive process furthers these goals.

Adaptation is the process of promoting total integrity. Integrity implies the soundness of an unimpaired condition leading to completeness and wholeness. Health, then, is a state and a process of being and becoming an integrated and whole person. Some people have found the notion of the health-illness continuum useful, yet it is a limited view and reflects a given point in time on a continuum. But because health is a dynamic concept, it is a process of being and becoming. In this sense whether the patient is a quadraplegic who carries out painting and writing poetry with mechanical devices or a person who uses drugs first to get through exams and then begins to be dependent on them, changes are evident in the individual's being and becoming integrated and whole.

These changes are entirely different than notions related to disease processes. By the same reasoning, dying individuals are going through that process of final being and becoming where they are integrating themselves. They have no immediate concern about their physical needs, if they are comfortable and can focus on integrating the self by considering personal accomplishments and satisfying their relationships with others. This can be the total integrating of the person and perhaps the very healthiest a person can be at that point in time.

NURSING

The last major element is nursing. According to the Roy model, nursing must first be considered in terms of goals. The goal of nursing is to promote adaptation by the use of the nursing process, in each of the adaptive modes, thus contributing to health, quality of life, and dying with dignity. The nurse states the adaptive or ineffective behavior with the most relevant influencing factor. Goals are set by looking at the first-level assessment and deciding with the patient what behavioral outcomes are expected from the plan for better integrating and adapting to his or her life. Interventions are the approaches used to manage the stimuli. Behavior is the result of the pooling of all these stimuli; nursing can examine these and intervene by helping the person manage the stimuli that are causing the adaptation. Evaluation is identifying the outcomes of interventions and judging whether they are effective in reaching the goal.

Thus far, this chapter has examined the assumptions of the Roy Adaptation Model, and the model's description of the four major concepts of person, environment, health, and nursing. These conceptual elements reflect the same themes as the assumptions of holism, mutuality, control processes, activity, creativity, purpose, and value. The knowledge necessary for nursing involves the processes by which persons positively affect their health in general. In the Roy model, these are the adaptive processes and the nursing actions to enhance these processes.

Research and
Practice Implications

The Roy Adaptation Model can direct practice and research. As a practice discipline, nursing focuses on nursing's function of promoting adaptation, that is, nursing diagnoses, interventions, and outcomes for persons or groups. Nursing as a practice discipline can be seen from the point of view of the role of the nurse. Model-based practice helps look at how nursing models are taught. It sheds light on the content of nursing. Implementing the model of nursing care in whole health care systems will require another area of expertise, both in implementation and in evaluation of the outcomes. Some of the outcomes are important in relation to what the model does for nursing, such as increasing autonomy, accountability, and professionalism in general, and in changing relationships with other disciplines.

Research based on the Roy model involves inquiry into basic life processes and how nursing enhances those processes. Research based on the model develops basic science, as well as a practice discipline. The research focuses on persons or groups adapting and on those adaptive processes that affect health status.

Given the advances of basic neurosciences, there is more known about the exquisite architecture of the cerebral cortex. Through technology one can observe the function of the human brain at work, when glucose molecules are tagged and viewed in action by nuclear magnetic resonance imaging. One can see a person processing language and music and making an association between the two. Nurse researchers, using the Roy Model, are putting together propositions related to the changes in physiological life processes and cognitive processing during brain injury; these highlight the neurochemical endocrine channels and also focus on the biorhythms of vulnerability, strength, and alterations in the neurotransmitters.

The aims of the first phase of research are to determine the direction and degree of change in these simultaneous and successive modes of processing—in particular in subjects with mild and moderate closed head injuries—and to determine the relationship between specific demographic and medical factors. The relevant factors are age, severity, social history, incidence of the pressures that are changing the processes, and the nature and degree of evident change. Cognitive recovery in relation to developing knowledge of vulnerable periods, neuroplasticity, and sensory input is being studied. The program of research focuses on descriptive and interventive studies of subjects with mild and moderate head injuries.

On a more global level, the primacy of the notion of integration, reflecting on holism, mutuality and control processes of the system, leads to the principle of "verativity," a term coined recently when speaking of values for science. It comes from the Latin word *veritas*, meaning truth. In the adaptive person, verativity reflects activity, creativity, unity, purpose, and value.

In summary, it is believed that, through continued insights from clinical practice, and with systematic sequential and often long and hard research efforts, scholars will continue to develop and disseminate nursing knowledge so that theoretical models can provide the bridge to excellence in practice.

REFERENCES

Andrews, H., and Roy, C. (1986). *Essentials of the Roy adaptation model.* Norwalk, CT: Appleton-Century-Crofts.

Donaldson, S. K., and Crowley, D. M. (1978). The discipline of nursing. *Nursing Outlook, 26* (2): 113-118.

Fawcett, J. (1984). *Analysis and evaluation of conceptual models of nursing.* Philadelphia: F. A. Davis Co.

Roy, C. (1976). *Introduction to nursing: An adaptation model.* Englewood Cliffs, NJ: Prentice-Hall.

Roy, C., and Roberts, S. (1981). *Theory construction in nursing: An adaptation model.* Englewood Cliffs, NJ: Prentice-Hall.

Roy, C. (1984). *Introduction to nursing: An adaptation model.* 2nd ed. Englewood Cliffs, NJ: Prentice-Hall.

4

A Critique of the Roy Adaptation Model

Mary H. Huch

Structure

HISTORICAL EVOLUTION

Roy's Adaptation Model evolved from work Roy undertook as a graduate student with encouragement from Dorothy Johnson. The writings of Helson (1964), a physiologist, provided the foundation for Roy's model. Early written presentations (Roy, 1970, 1971) included most of the assumptions now explicitly stated in her work. According to Roy (1970), the model provides for the development of three postulates, namely, adaptation problems, coping mechanisms, and nursing intervention. Each proposed postulate is directed toward some aspect of the adaptive process for the observation and classification of phenomena. The purpose of the adaptive problem's postulate is to delineate the range of possible responses of a person along the health-illness continuum. Two coping mechanisms, cognator and regulator, are identified and explained. The cognator subsystem involves the mental and emotional processes used by a person to adapt. The regulator subsystem includes the physiological responses called into play in a situation requiring adaptation (Roy and Roberts, 1981). Both of these mechanisms have four modes whereby adaptation occurs: physiologic needs, self-concept, role function, and interdependence.

The interrelationship of the coping mechanisms and modes of adaptation may be more easily understood by further explanation. When some stimulus impinges on an individual, a series of events takes place. First, there is arousal of the cognator and regulator subsystems. In turn, the four adaptive modes are set into action to function as effectors of adaptation. It is possible for some events to involve more than one of the modes simultaneously. Through this process, adaptive or ineffective responses occur (Roy and McLeod, 1981). The nursing intervention postulate is to provide the basis for decision making in the provision of nursing care. These proposed ideas for postulate formulation are foundational to the development of a nursing science. Knowledge that unfolds in the development of the Roy Adaptation Model is envisioned as the basis for nursing curricula, nursing practice, and nursing research (Roy, 1970).

From the beginning, the Roy Adaptation Model has continued to evolve to the stage where assumptions underlying the model are explicitly stated and additional assumptions are developing. These assumptions begin with the nature of Man and progress through the process of adapting.

PHILOSOPHICAL ASSUMPTIONS

Each of the eight basic assumptions will be explored to provide further insight for understanding the structure of the model.

Assumption 1.

"The person is a bio-psycho-social being" (Roy, 1980, p. 180). The person is viewed from a variety of perspectives that address the biological, psychological, and social aspects.

Assumption 2.

"The person is in constant interaction with a changing environment" (Roy, 1980, p. 180). The multifaceted person described in the first assumption is in continual interaction with the environment, which has an everchanging, dynamic quality. Resulting from the need for continual readjusting, the person must have some means to maintain a measure of equilibrium.

Assumption 3.

"To cope with a changing world, the person uses both innate and acquired mechanisms, which are biologic, psychologic, and social in origin" (Roy, 1980, p. 180). This provides the means for readjustment. The person has the ability to use mechanisms that occur naturally and those that must be learned.

Assumption 4.

"Health and illness are one inevitable dimension of life" (Roy, 1980, p. 181). The person exists along a health-illness continuum. This fourth assumption indicates there are degrees of wellness that can be obtained.

Assumption 5.

"To respond positively to environmental changes, the person must adapt" (Roy 1980, p. 181). This brings into play the adaptation process. The person is best served by a positive response to the everchanging environment.

Assumption 6.

"The person's adaptation is a function of the stimulus he is exposed to and his adaptation level" (Roy, 1980, p. 181). The stimulus may be one of three types. The first, focal in nature, is one that immediately has an impact on the person. The second consists of contextual stimuli: interrelated events occurring simultaneously with the focal stimuli. Residual is the third type of stimuli. The residual stimuli come from within the person and reflect attitudes, beliefs, and values. Specific attitudes, beliefs, and values come into play only if they have an effect on the situation being examined.

Assumption 7.

"The person's adaptation level is such that it comprises a zone indicating the range of stimulation that will lead to a positive response" (Roy, 1980, p. 181). This provides a means of determining the magnitude of a stimulus needed for a positive response. It is through a positive response that adaptation occurs. The positive adaptation may occur by means of the four modes.

Assumption 8.

"The person is conceptualized as having four modes of adaptation: physiologic needs, self-concept, role function, and interdependence relations" (Roy, 1980, p. 182). These eight assumptions serve as the basis for the Roy Adaptation Model.

More recent writings have focused on systems and on viewing the person as an adaptive system. Though this scientific structure is used, there is a concomitant emphasis on the person as a holistic being. Nursing has a humanistic basis and as such accepts the views and beliefs of other persons (Roy, 1984). Likewise, the concept of health is not only a state but also a process. It is through this process that an individual becomes an integrated, whole person (Roy, 1984). These assumptions have been added to the eight from previous writings to bring about a more humanistic focus.

PRINCIPLES, CONCEPTS, AND PROPOSITIONS

Throughout Roy's presentation of the Adaptation Model, no principles are explicitly stated. The two subsystems (cognator and regulator) and their four modes (physiologic needs, self-concept, role function, and interdependence relations) provide the concepts of the model. Internal and external stimuli are responsible for activating each of the subsystems. The resulting response occurs directionally with the ultimate outcome being adaptation or a nonadaptive state called ineffective adaptation.

An example of a specific directional proposition of the regulator subsystem is "intact neural pathways will positively influence neural output to effectors" (Roy and McLeod, 1981, p. 62). Similarly, the cognator subsystem has directional propositions with one such being "the higher the level of adequacy of all the cognator processes, the more effective the psychomotor choice of response" (Roy and McLeod, 1981, p. 65). Roy wrote that the regulator subsystem is linked primarily to the physiologic needs mode of adaptation, leading to the conclusion that the cognator subsystem is more closely linked with the self-concept, role function, and interdependence relations modes.

Though a separate series of propositions is developed for each of the modes linked to the cognator subsystem, no separate set of propositions has been developed for the physiologic needs mode. Physiologic needs are discussed in relation to the propositions of the regulator subsystem (Roy and Roberts, 1981). This presents a situation of semantic incongruity. If in fact the four modes are the manifestation of regulator and cognator activity (Roy and McLeod, 1981), the propositions of these two subsystems should be sufficient for delineating the relationships of the concepts.

DEFINITION OF MAN

Man is defined as a bio-psycho-social being. Such a perspective indicates that Man can be parceled into separate components for analysis and study. This creates the illusion of dealing with separate parts of Man. If one is viewed as having separate parts or components, it is much easier to take care of an apparent problem without viewing the whole. For example, a young child falls, injures a leg, and is brought to a health care agency for treatment. The nurse provides expert care in treating the leg injury. Unfortunately, the circumstances surrounding the injury are not investigated. This child has been struggling with the addition of a new sibling and has been acting out by taking many risks in playtime activities in order to attract the mother's attention. The leg was injured in one of these risk-taking adventures. Further exploration of Roy's concept of Man as a bio-psycho-social being does present the idea that Man is a unified whole to be examined from biological, psychological, and sociological components. Accordingly, Man is viewed by Roy as "a whole made up of parts or subsystems that function as a unity for some purpose" (Roy and McLeod, 1981, p. 53).

The concept of wholeness is more than the addition of the subparts. Unity implies a oneness that cannot be understood by separating the subparts. The subparts do not give a full understanding of the whole being. To view the component parts of Man as an additive function presents Man as a mechanistic being, much as various pieces are put together to make a dress, a chair, or a motor. Man as a person is the central focus of the model (Roy, 1970, 1980). Family, community, and society as a focus of nursing care was enunciated in the work of Roy and Roberts (1981) and Roy (1984).

This conception of Man at first glance seems to be somewhat simplistic and straightforward. Roy's eight assumptions undergird the model. Definitions are provided for key terms. The interrelationship of some of the concepts is not clear. Specifically, propositions are developed for the cognator and regulator subsystems. Yet the process of responding seems to occur independently within each of these subsystems as presented. "The regulator subsystem is related predominately to the mode of physiologic needs" (Roy and McLeod, 1981, p. 67). Roy and McLeod (1981) wrote that perception is the link between the cognator and regulator. Such a relationship between the two subsystems is not clearly evident within the presentation. In fact, Roy and McLeod (1981) wrote that, "Since very little is known physiologically about the process of perception formation, memory, and choice of psychomotor responses, the other modes of self-concept, role function, and interdependence must relate to the meaning of a given perception for the individual human system" (p. 67).

Further exploration of the model shows Man is a complex being made even more so by the constant interaction with changing environment (Roy, 1980). As Roy further refined the model within the context of systems theory, an explicit statement is made that "the nursing model directs that the nurse view the patient holistically" (Roy and McLeod, 1981, p. 49). The person, however, is described as an adaptive system. Man initially responds to a variety of internal and external stimuli. For each person, there exists a variable standard that is that person's adaptation level. The adaptation level is affected by focal, contextual, and residual stimuli (Roy, 1980). Through the process of adaptation, Man is able to adjust to the stimuli impinging from the environment. Man is acted upon by the environment and responds to the environment by adapting. Having this ability, Man contributes toward the meeting of health goals. Through effective adaptation, energy is freed. The freeing of energy provides the resource for use in attaining health (Roy, 1981).

DEFINITION OF HEALTH

Health is presented as the opposite of illness, and an individual may be located at any point on the health-illness continuum (Roy, 1970, 1980). The individual uses adaptation as a means of responding to environmental stimuli, that in turn causes needs to arise. Successful adaptation indicates that a positive response to an environmental stimulus has occurred (Roy, 1980). This is an example of linear causality. When successful adaptation occurs, a healthful state exists. The concept of health is defined by Roy (1984) as "a state and a process of being and becoming an integrated and whole person" (p. 39). This definition is incongruous with the previous conception of health as a state along a continuum. Now, health is not only a state but also "a process of being and becoming" (Roy, 1984, p. 39). The previous linear perspective of health is being moved toward a more unified conceptualization of Man and being, yet this new definition remains inconsistent with the model itself. Being and becoming have meanings that are incongruent with the causal grounding of Man as an adaptive organism.

Some additional terms quite consistent with Roy's Model (for example, high-level wellness and peak wellness, Roy, 1980) have been used. These additional terms are not defined in this nor subsequent writings. These and similar terms are used as identified points along the health-illness continuum. There is no quantification of what is missing from normal health that will produce poor health. Though there continues to be an emphasis on striving toward high-level wellness, there has been no further move to more clearly differentiate these terms.

RELATIONSHIP BETWEEN MAN AND HEALTH

An integral part of the concept of health is the adaptive response in Man. Roy and McLeod (1981) have stated:

The person encounters adaptation problems in changing environments, especially in situations of health and illness. These problems are the concern of the nurse and her goal will be to solve the problem and bring about adaptation. . . . This goal provides a conceptual basis for deciding whether or not a person needs nursing. (p. 45)

This statement suggests a one-way relationship on the part of the nurse. The nurse is "to solve the problem and bring about adaptation" (Roy and McLeod 1981, p. 45); there is no indication that the individual takes an active role in the decision-making process.

As the nurse interacts with the patient, means are sought whereby ineffective responses can be overcome. To achieve the end of determining whether a response is effective or ineffective, the nurse begins with a first-level assessment. For this process, data are gathered and categorized relative to each of the four adaptive modes. Interviewing, observing, and measuring of responses are the methods of data collection. A tentative judgment of ineffective responses is made by the nurse and patient. Roy (1984) identified criteria used in making this judgment as "whether or not the behavior promotes integrity of the individual, whether or not there is regulator and cognator effectiveness, and whether or not the person perceives the behavior as adaptive" (p. 51). As the ineffective responses are ameliorated, a higher level of health ensues.

A person is constantly interacting with a changing environment. The impact of environmental stimuli causes the development of needs within the individual. The person being stimulated will try to maintain the integrity of being through adaptation. The nursing adaptation process occurs through the use of four modes (physiological needs, self-concept, role function, and interdependence) related to the cognator and regulator subsystems. Each mode can be related to one of the components of Man's nature; this is, physiological needs relate to the biological component; self-concept relates to the psychological component; and role function and interdependence relate to the sociological component. This is a reductionistic approach. As a result of Man's response to environmental stimuli in a positive manner, adaptation takes place and some degree of health is attained. From this description of the model, it can be readily seen that, according to Roy (1984), Man exists in varying states of health ranging from optimal health to maximal illness or death. The latest published definition of health is incongruent with the model itself.

The nurse is needed "when unusual stresses or weakened coping mechanisms make usual attempts to cope ineffective" (Roy and Roberts, 1981, p. 45). The nurse assesses the four modes of adapting and, based on the data obtained from the assessment, determines which behaviors are ineffective and which are adaptive. For ineffective behaviors (diminished health state), a second-level of assessment is undertaken to identify focal, contextual, and residual stimuli impinging upon the individual. The nurse sets the direction for this aspect of the assessment, although the patient should "be involved in every phase of the plan of care" (Roy, 1984, p. 52). Following the data-gathering process and validation of effector stimuli, a nursing diagnosis is stated. Based on the diagnosis the appropriate nursing interventions are then determined and "the nurse acts as an external regulatory force to modify stimuli affecting adaptation" (Roy, 1980, p. 186). In this manner an individual is assisted to an improved health state. With the nurse setting the direction for assessment, the person's influence in decision making can be diminished.

Process

CORRESPONDENCE

Established Knowledge of Man and Health

Roy wrote of Man as a being having multiple dimensions or components. This bio-psycho-social being is seen as being "in constant interaction with a changing environment" (Roy, 1970; Roy 1980). Adaptation is the means by which Man sustains health. As needs are exhibited, attempts are made to alter the stimuli causing the need.

As internal and external environments change, the level of satiety for any need changes. When satiety changes, then a deficit or excess is created. This deficit or excess triggers off the appropriate adaptive mode. (Roy, 1980, p. 184)

This approach for the understanding of Man and relationship of Man and health as dynamic interaction has been enunciated by at least one other nurse theorist, namely, King (1981), who wrote that:

Health is a dynamic state in the life cycle of a human being, which implies continuous adjustment to stressors in the internal and external environment through optimum use of one's resources to achieve maximum potential for daily living. (p. 5)

The complexity of Man is dealt with by viewing Man "as having parts or elements linked together in such a way that force on the linkage can be increased or decreased" (Roy, 1980, p. 179). Though there are elements or parts, Man, according to Roy, does function as a unified being. This approach fits well with commonly accepted beliefs.

In contrast to Roy's belief, other nurse scholars have conceived of Man as a unitary being. Rogers (1970) wrote that Man is unitary in nature. Parse (1981), like Rogers, has posited that "Man is synergistic, more than and different from the sum of parts. . . . Man, unified, can be recognized through individual patterns of relating." (p. 28) These theorists provide support for the concept that Man is more than and different from the sum of parts, unlike Roy who views Man as a composite of the individual parts.

Health as a state of being with varying degrees of wellness is frequently found in the literature. Dunn (1973) wrote of high-level wellness and its achievement, and postulated that wellness has varying degrees or levels:

High level wellness for the individual is defined as an integrated method of functioning which is oriented toward maximizing the potential of which the individual is capable. It requires that the individual maintain a continuum of balance and purposeful direction within the environment where he is functioning. (pp. 4-5)

Numerous schools of nursing are using the health-illness continuum as part of the organizing structure for the curriculum. Orem (1985) wrote about the classification of nursing situations that are differentiated based on a level of wellness or health. Clearly, Roy's Adaptation Model fits well with the established general knowledge about Man and health as explicated in the well-known traditional medical model as practiced in nursing.

Interrelation of Concepts at Same Level of Discourse

There seem to be two sets of concepts in the Roy Model. The subsystems cognator and regulator make up one set. These are written at the same level of discourse. The second set of concepts, the modes of adaptation, vary in level of discourse. The term physiological is not at the same language level with self-concept, role function, and interdependence. Terms such as psychological and sociological are consistent with physiological and could be used to refer to self-concept, role function, and interdependence, respectively.

Relationship to Paradigmatic Perspectives and Philosophical Assumptions

Roy's model is a clear example of a theory in the totality paradigm (Parse and others, 1985). In the totality paradigm, Man is viewed as bio-psycho-social-spiritual being adapting to the environment. Health is a point on a continuum and can be changed through the intervention of health care providers. The totality paradigm is in stark contrast to the simultaneity paradigm (Parse and others, 1985). In the latter, Man is an open system in mutual interaction with the environment, and has responsibility and chooses a course of action. Within the simultaneity paradigm, health is viewed as a process of becoming rather than a state and process of adaptation.

Description and Meaning of Principles, Concepts and Propositions

Throughout the writings of Roy, the individual concepts are readily understood. As there are no principles stated as such, there can be some difficulty in understanding how some of the concepts fit together to fully comprehend the model. A good example involves the cognator and regular subsystems, originally called mechanisms (Roy, 1970), and the four adaptive modes (Roy, 1971). These early writings provided no linkage between the subsystem (mechanism) and adaptive modes. Roy (1980) indicated "the assumption that the person has four modes of adaptation" (p. 188) should be validated. Yet the concepts of cognator and regulator are not addressed within this presentation of the model. In Roy and McLeod (1981), the relationship between regulator and cognator and the four adaptive modes is made clearer. A possible reason for some of the lack of clarity in the relationship of these concepts comes from Roy (1984) who in 1984 wrote that "the theoretical work on cognator and regulator processes is still in the beginning stages" (p. 35).

The impetus for the central concept of the model was derived from writings outside the discipline of nursing. Helson's work as a physiological psychologist focuses on neurological and psychological phenomena. Over time there has been a delineation of the model into a systems theory structure (Roy and Roberts, 1981), while continuing the strong focus on neurological-psychological functioning in mind-body dichotomy. The propositions of the regulator subsystem are primarily involved with neural activity which evidences this focus. The cognator subsystem focuses on functions of the mind.

The systems approach is well suited for the basic assumptions of the Roy Adaptation Model. The concepts of Man interacting with the environment and responding to internal and external stimuli is congruent with input into a system. Throughput occurs as a result of primary (regulator and cognator) and secondary (physiologic needs, self-concept, role function, and interdependence) subsystems leading to output, which can be the adaptive or ineffective responses. Both responses provide the feedback to the system so that the individual continually attempts to reach dynamic equilibrium. The person attempts to consistently move to a higher level of wellness. Wellness is addressed in relation to the effectiveness of adaptive responses. Effective responses are "those that promote the integrity of the person in terms of goals of the person-system, survival, growth, reproduction, and mastery" (Roy, 1984, p. 49).

Each successive publication of Roy's model has more clearly described its concepts. The previously used example of cognator and regulator subsystems serves well to show an increasing attention to some concepts. While the first writing of Roy (1970) briefly presented and explained these concepts, Roy and McLeod (1981) presented a fairly extensive list of propositions related to the cognator and regulator subsystems. At no time has there been an "invention" of words or the use of words in a way not readily discernible by the audience to whom the writing is addressed. Roy's Adaptation Model clearly flows from the writings of Helson (1964) on the concept of adaptation. With such an understandable approach to presentation of the concepts, the model becomes a good candidate for use in both practice and educational settings. Though there are a number of key words used in the model, the greatest portion are easily understood in and of themselves. The individual first approaching the model can profit from further clarification of concepts such as regulator subsystem, cognator subsystem, and adaptation level.

Overall, these terms are explained in more recent writings and are understandable. Related key terms are semantically inconsistent. Most pointedly the inconsistency is seen in the four adaptive modes. The self-concept, role function, and interdependence modes are grouped together by Roy (1984) as psychosocial adaptive modes. Some consistency could be achieved with one important change. Self-concept, role function, and interdependence should be functions or aspects of a generalized mode rather than being considered as separate modes. Such a perspective provides for consistency of language. Roy (1981) did specify propositions that show the relationship of subconcepts within each of the four adaptive modes, written in directional terms to show cause-effect relationships. An example from the self-concept mode is: "The numbers of social rewards positively influence the quantity of social experience" (p. 225). The language level is appropriate and the syntax is consistent with the totality paradigm.

COHERENCE

Relation of Model to Other Theories

Roy's Adaptation Model clearly flows from the work of Helson. The concepts of focal, contextual, and residual stimuli are directly attributable to him and serve as key elements during the second level of assessment. The extent of Helson's influence is most apparent in Roy and Robert's book *Theory Construction in Nursing: An Adaptation Model*.

Some aspects of the model are similar to the concepts of other theories/frameworks. More particularly, Roy's concept of Man as an integrated "whole made up of parts or subsystems that function as a unity for some purpose" (Roy and McLeod, 1981, p. 53) has been espoused by other theorists.

The work of Johnson (1980) has also presented the concept of Man functioning with parts comprising the whole: "Although each subsystem has a specialized task or function, the system as a whole depends upon an integrated performance" (p. 210). She further posited that:

The subsystems and the system as a whole tend to be self-maintaining and self-perpetuating so long as the condition in the internal and external environment of the system remain orderly and predictable, the conditions and resources necessary to their functional requirements are met, and the interrelationships among the subsystems are harmonious. (p. 212)

This perspective implies a dynamic state with movement to maintain balance or to achieve some level of functioning.

Roy (1980) wrote of the person's use of innate and acquired mechanisms to cope while constantly interacting with the environment. Again, one finds an explicit statement indicative of movement and change occurring with Man. In more recent development of the model, Roy posited "there is a dynamic objective for human existence with the ultimate goal of achieving dignity and integrity" (Roy, 1984, p. 38).

Logical Flow from Assumptions to Propositions

The assumptions of the Roy Adaptation Model progress in an orderly fashion. The central focus of the model is identified as the person and the first assumption of the model is "the person is a bio-psycho-social being" (Roy, 1980, p. 180). From this point the assumptions progress to include the role of the environment (changing), origin of coping mechanisms (innate and acquired), categorization of stimuli for change (focal, contextual, and residual), the modes of adaptation (physiologic needs, self-concept, role function, and interdependence) (Roy, 1970; Roy, 1980) and use of a humanistic approach to nursing (Roy, 1984). It has been stated explicitly by Roy that "the Roy Adaptation Model can be viewed primarily as a systems model" (Roy, 1980, p. 179). The model can be classified in this way, and the components of the model easily fit a systems approach.

Using a systems model, Roy and McLeod (1981) developed a theory of the person as an adaptive system. Stimuli from within and outside the person, also called stressors, serve as the input to the system. The two subsystems, regulator and cognator, are aroused in response to the stimuli. The regulator subsystem is involved in physiological responses to the stimuli, while the cognator subsystem is involved with cognitive and emotional responses to stimuli. These two subsystems, along with their four adaptive modes, provide for the throughput of the system. The output results from the adaptive activity and is manifested as an adaptive or ineffective response. Either or both of these responses serve as the feedback mechanisms. Rather than the theory of the person as an adaptive system being a move toward a general system theory, it fits more readily as a body systems approach to the understanding of human function.

The recent addition of humanistic values to the provision of nursing care adds warmth and caring to what could be conceived of as a purely physiological, behavioral view of Man. This increased dimension of the model is especially valuable with the tremendous emphasis today on high technology in the provision of health care. The quality of valuing a person and striving for dignity and integrity bring forth "high touch" to the technology world. Yet these assumptions do not ground the theory; in fact, they create a semantic gap. For example, one assumption is that nurses use a holistic approach in the care of patients (Roy, 1984). Review of the theory of a person as an adaptive system shows this assumption is not included in the discussion. The whole of the adaptive process is very mechanistic. The assumptions do flow, one from the other, in a progressive manner except for the more recent addition of the explicit statement about humanistic values. This creates an obvious structural addition to the model, which is clearly not integrated. Without the humanistic assumptions, the logical sequence is readily discernible.

Symmetry and Aesthetics

With the Roy model, the individual parts are used to organize the whole in a symmetrical way. Balance is achieved by the horizontal flow of action and subsequent feedback mechanism of a systems approach. The model can be considered generally aesthetic in presentation.

PRAGMATICS

Use of Model in Practice and Research

From her earliest writings, Roy has promulgated the Adaptation Model as a basis for nursing practice (1971). The neuropsychological influence in the model's development contributes to its utility in the medical model practice arena. Starr (1980) applied the Roy Adaptation Model to the care of a dying patient, and Schmitz (1980) provided a very detailed application of the model to the care of a patient in a community setting. A very comprehensive presentation of application of the model in practice settings has been undertaken by Randell and others (1982). Some topics included are pediatric surgery, anxiety in the emergency room, chronic illness, a postnatal experience, depression and loss, and a child with a developmental delay. In each of these instances, Roy's Adaptation Model serves as the basis for providing traditional nursing care. It has been useful in supporting the traditional concept of nursing practice within the medical model perspective. The examples above encompass use of the nursing process with an adaptation focus and its application in a variety of settings. The nursing process is the basis of practice with the Roy Adaptation Model. No practice methodology has evolved from the model; the practice is articulated as the all-inclusive nursing process, which does not have its ontological base in Roy's model.

The model is based on theoretical formulations developed in another discipline (Helson, 1964). Nonetheless, some nurse researchers have attempted to provide empirical data for support of the model. Fawcett (1981), Idle (1978), and Lewis and others (1979) are just a few who have attempted to validate the theory through research. Roy and McLeod (1981) set forth numerous examples of hypotheses for practice. They wrote, "one important function of theory is to generate testable hypotheses for research" (p. 257). Research is the means for joining theory and practice. Yet, within the references listed, little if any nursing research is indicated in support of the suggested hypotheses.

The model is used extensively in nursing education. Its use even extends beyond the United States and includes Canada and Switzerland. As of 1982, a total of 27 schools of nursing were using the model (Fawcett, 1984). By using the model as a basis for curriculum development, there is a greater likelihood of developing nurses who use the model within their nursing practice. It does, however, sustain the practice of nursing within the traditional medical model framework.

Guidelines for practice emanate from the model, and further explication of concepts can take place through research. Research is the area that needs increased emphasis so that there can be clearer delineation of the four adaptive modes and the appropriate nursing interventions.

Contribution to Nursing Science

In 1970 Roy wrote "the adaptation model provides a conceptual framework for nursing. Such a framework may be the basis for developing a nursing science . . ." (p. 45). Roy has provided a significant contribution to nursing knowledge through provisions of a framework for education, practice, and research. In order that nursing can fully develop as a science, it is necessary to develop that knowledge which is unique to the discipline. Such will occur only through extensive research. It is in repeatedly deriving the same findings in similar situations that general laws will develop, and nursing will truly be a science. Roy has provided a firm foundation. Now it is imperative to further explicate the model's concepts through research.

REFERENCES

Dunn, H. L. (1973). *High-level wellness*. Arlington, VA: Beatty.

Fawcett, J. (1981). Needs of caesarean birth parents. *Journal of Obstetric, Gynecologic, and Neonatal Nursing, 10*:371-376.

Fawcett, J. (1984). *Analysis and evaluation of conceptual models of nursing*. Philadelphia, F. A. Davis Co.

Helson, H. (1964). *Adaptation level theory*. New York: Harper & Row.

Idle, B. A. (1978), SPAL: A tool for measuring self-perceived adaptation level appropriate for an elderly population. *In* E. E. Bauwens ed., *Clinical nursing research: Its strategies and findings*. Indianapolis: Sigma Theta Tau.

Johnson, D. E. (1980). The behavioral system model for nursing. *In* J. P. Riehl and C. Roy, eds., *Conceptual models for nursing*.

King, I. M. (1981). *A theory for nursing: Systems, concepts, process*. New York: John Wiley & Sons.

Lewis, F. M., Firsich, S. C., and Parsell, S. (1979). Clinical tool development for adult chemotherapy patients: Process and content. *Cancer Nursing, 2*(2):99-108.

Nursing Development Conference Group (1979). *Concept formalization in nursing: Process and product*, 2nd ed. Boston: Little, Brown and Company.

Orem, D. E. (1985). *Nursing: Concepts of practice*, 3rd ed. New York: McGraw-Hill Book Co.

Parse, R. R. (1981). *Man-living-health: A theory of nursing*. New York: John Wiley & Sons.

Parse, R. R., Coyne, A. B., and Smith, M. J. (1985). *Nursing research: Qualitative methods*. Bowie, MD: Brady Communications.

Randell, B., Poush Tedrow, M., and Van Landingham, J. (1982). *Adaptation Nursing: The Roy conceptual model applied*. St. Louis: C. V. Mosby Co.

Rogers, M. E. (1970). *An Introduction to the theoretical basis of nursing*. Philadelphia: F. A. Davis Co.

Roy, C. (1970). Adaptation: A conceptual framework for nursing. *Nursing Outlook, 18*(3):42-45.

Roy, C. (1971). Adaptation: A basis for nursing practice. *Nursing Outlook, 19*(4):254-257.

Roy, C. (1973). Adaptation: Implications for curriculum change. *Nursing Outlook, 21*(3):163-168.

Roy, C. (1980). The Roy adaptation model. *In* J. P. Riehl and C. Roy, eds. *Conceptual models for nursing practice*. New York: Appleton-Century-Crofts.

Roy, C. (1984). *Introduction to nursing: An adaptation model*. Englewood Cliffs, NJ: Prentice-Hall.

Roy, C., and McLeod, D. (1981). Theory of the person as an adaptive system. *In* C. Roy and S. L. Roberts, *Theory construction in nursing: An adaptation model*. Englewood Cliffs, NJ: Prentice-Hall.

Roy, C., and Roberts, S. L. (1981). *Theory construction in nursing: An adaptation model*. Englewood Cliffs, NJ: Prentice-Hall.

Schmitz, M. (1980). The Roy adaptation model: Application in a community
    setting. *In* J. P. Riehl and C. Roy, eds, *Conceptual models for nursing prac-
    tice,* 2nd ed. New York: Appleton-Century-Crofts.
Starr, S. L. (1980). Adaptation applied to the dying client. *In* J. P. Riehl and C.
    Roy, eds, *Conceptual models for nursing practice,* 2nd ed. New York: Ap-
    pleton-Century-Crofts.

5

Orem's General Theory of Nursing

DOROTHEA E. OREM

EDITORIAL PERSPECTIVE

Orem (1985) describes Man as an organism that has self-care capabilities. The capabilities are physical, psychological, social, and spiritual aspects. This view of Man is consistent with the totality paradigm. Orem (1985) has defined health as a dynamic state of well-being, which is consistent with the totality paradigm view that health is a state, on a continuum with non health. Orem differs from Roy (1984) in that Roy stays within medical science to specify her nursing model. The language of Roy's model gives evidence of this. The language of Orem's theory is not the language of medical science, but rather a general theory of nursing formalized as a triad of theories.

On the following pages, Orem (1985) specifically discusses the emergence of her general theory of nursing. She explains

67

the meaning of various terms used in the theory as well as her
views about Man and health.

Since 1958, the writer has been involved in inquiry into the
question, What is the domain and what are the boundaries of nursing as a field of knowledge and a field of practice? One result of
this endeavor has the form of an expressed general conceptualization or theory of nursing, the self-care deficit theory, with its distinctive conceptual structure. The articulated concepts of the theory
identify the elements of the domain of nursing and provide a basis
for making inferences about nursing's boundaries. The broad concepts of this general theory of nursing and the underlying structure
of the concepts provide points of articulation of nursing with other
fields of knowledge and other fields of practical endeavor including
the health services. The dynamic state of development of the underlying structure of broad concepts of the theory is "fruitful in the
isolation of research methodologies of nursing" (Nursing Development Conference Group, 1979, p. 130).

The insights about nursing expressed in 1979 as a general
theory of nursing were attained over a period of more than 20
years. The understanding of nursing as a field of knowledge and
practice have resulted from solitary work, work with graduate students in the School of Nursing of the Catholic University of America (CUA), work with colleagues on CUA's Committee on the
Nursing Model, and work with colleagues in the Nursing Development Conference Group. Work with educators in nursing and with
nursing practitioners and researchers in the United States and Canada has contributed in a major way to the continued development
of a general theory of nursing. Some results of these endeavors
are recorded in *Nursing: Concepts of Practice* (3rd ed., 1985), *in
Concept Formalization in Nursing: Process and Product* (2nd ed.,
1979), and in prior editions of both books.

A System of Concepts

The self-care deficit theory of nursing is constituted from a core of related concepts and from peripheral but related concepts. The core concepts are associated with the person elements of nursing practice situations, namely, legitimate nurse and legitimate patient (Nursing Development Conference Group, 1979, p. 168). The sets of concepts associated with legitimate patient include: self-care, self-care agency, therapeutic self-care demand, and self-care deficit, which is a relational concept. The set of concepts associated with legitimate nurse include nursing agency and nursing system, that is, the action system through which nursing results are achieved. Peripheral concepts include those within the complex conceptual construct named basic conditioning factors, that is, factors that are determinants of the qualitative or quantitative characteristics of elements of the core concepts as they are identified in concrete situations of nursing practice.

The core concepts, with the exception of nursing system, are represented in Figure 5-1. The core of articulated concepts named in the figure form a relatively simple structure. The conceptual elements represent formulated and expressed insights and judgments about the unity in the concrete individuality of data obtained from nursing practice situations. In its broadest sense the conceptual system represents judgments about a singular combination of properties of persons who require nursing and of nurses common to all situations of nursing practice. It is not an explanation of the individuality of any one situation. The relative simplicity of the conceptual system expressed in the late 1970s (six core concepts and one peripheral concept) is evident when contrasted with an earlier representation (Orem, 1959, p. 21) of nursing elements shown in Figure 5-2.

The conceptual system is the expression of the meaning of features of nursing practice situations (Wallace, 1979, p. 44; Nursing Development Conference Group, 1979, pp. 129-180). The terms used to express the concepts of the system are presented in Appendix A; explanatory terms are differentiated from experiential terms. According to Lonergan (1958, pp. 80-81), experiential terms are verified in terms of combinations of experiences. For

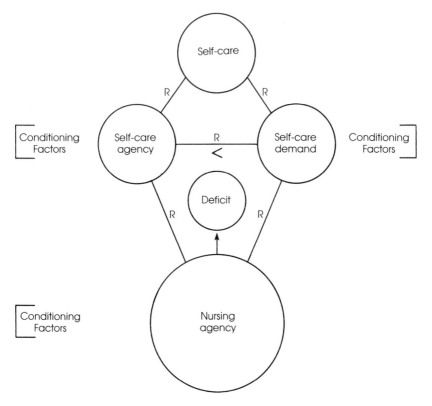

FIGURE 5-1
Conceptual structure of the self-care deficit theory of nursing.

example, eating, as an aspect of self-care, is an experiential term
while self-care is an explanatory term.

The conceptual system represented in Figure 5-1 had its beginning in an understanding that provided the writer with the answer to the question, Why do human beings require nursing? A
valid answer would name the human condition as the specific concern of nurses. The condition began to be understood in 1958 as
the health-derived or health-related inability of persons to provide
continuously for themselves the required quality and quantity of
self-care. In those nursing situations involving children or other dependents and their care agents, the health-care requirements of

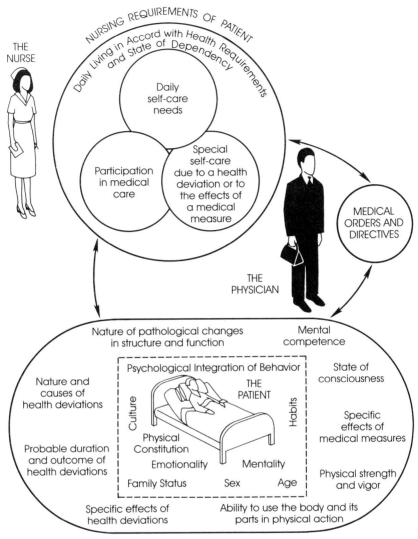

FIGURE 5-2
Nursing the patient: frameworks for nursing action.

the dependent persons were understood as the reason for the limitation of the care agent (Orem, 1985, pp. 18–19).

The conceptual system also has foundations in the acceptance that nursing is a human health service with the attendant understanding that nursing is a form of practical endeavor. This leads to the acceptance that nursing knowledge has the form of a practice discipline or a practical science (Wallace, 1959, pp. 263-274).

The broad essential concepts of the self-care deficit theory of nursing give meaning and structure to a range of phenomena in concrete situations of nursing practice. The conceptual system as a whole and the theories of which the concepts are parts are viewed as descriptively explanatory of nursing. If one does not accept that nursing is a practical endeavor of nurses that seeks results beneficial to others and that there is a human condition with which nurses deal as nurses, there is no basis for accepting this theoretical system that affords meaning to nursing.

A Triad of Articulated Theories

Increased understanding of the conceptual system described in the foregoing section enabled the writer in 1979 to elaborate three theories—self-care, self-care deficit, and nursing system. Together, in their articulations, these three theories are viewed as constituting a general theory of nursing. The theory of self-care deficit proposes an answer to the question, When and why do people require the health service nursing? The theory of self-care proposes an answer to the question, What is self-care and what is dependent care? The theory of nursing system proposes an answer to three questions: What do nurses do when they nurse? What is the product made by nurses? What results are sought by nurses? Each theory is expressed in terms of its central idea, a set of propositions, and set(s) of presuppositions (Orem, 1985, pp. 33-39).

PROCEDURE

The modes of procedure for formulating and expressing this general theory of nursing should be understood as both analytical and compositive. Analytical and compositive modes of procedure are used in practice disciplines (Wallace, 1979, pp. 269-274).

The expression of the three theories and their conceptual elements involved the use of a modeling technique using elements of deliberate human action including models of consciously coordinated actions of two or more persons. Models of deliberate action were linked to a wide range of models from nursing-related fields.

The terms used to name the concepts reflect the language of action theory. Literature used in the study of action theory included works of Aristotle and Thomas Aquinas, as well as modern works by logicians, philosophers, psychologists, physiologists, sociologists, and industrialists. Louise Hartnett Rauckhorst's conceptualization of voluntary human action involving motor activity exemplifies one type of model (Nursing Development Conference Group, 1979, pp. 135-141). The use of Parson's concept of the "unit action" from his elements of social action resulted in another type of model. This model set forth the action features of nursing situations (Nursing Development Conference Group, 1979, pp. 156-169, esp. p. 158).

ASSUMPTIONS

The general theory of nursing was elaborated and then formalized as a triad of theories in light of five assumptions about self-evident characteristics of human beings:

1. Human beings require continuous deliberate inputs to themselves and their environments in order to remain alive and to function in accord with natural human endowments.

2. Human agency, the power to act deliberately, is exercised in the form of care of self and others in identifying needs for self and others in making needed inputs.

3. Mature human beings experience privations in the form of limitations for action in care of self and others involving the making of life-sustaining and function-regulating inputs.

4. Human agency is exercised in discovering, developing, and transmitting to others ways and means to identify needs for self and others and make inputs to self and others.

5. Groups of human beings with structured relationships cluster tasks and allocate responsibilities for providing care to group members who experience privations for making required deliberate input to self and others.

The five assumptions about human characteristics were first expressed in 1973 in a paper titled "A General Theory of Nursing," presented at the Fifth Annual Post-masters Conference of Marquette University's School of Nursing. In the paper the five human characteristics were identified as "principles of nursing." Prior to 1973 the five assumptions were implicit in this writer's thinking but were not formally expressed.

It should be noted from the example given that the assumptions are expressed as propositions that pertain to ordinary experience. As propositions they make affirmations about the primitive characteristics of human beings. These assumptions are not theoretical, as they result from judgments of fact. They also are outside the realm of common sense, which deals with particular instances, not with generalizations. Whether they should be referred to as assumptions or principles is still to be answered. From this writer's perspective in theory formulation, they served as assumed empirical generalizations about human beings.

RELATION WITHIN THE TRIAD OF THEORIES

The theory of nursing system is the unifying theory within the triad and justifies reference to the three theories in their articulations as a general theory of nursing. The theory of self-care deficit or dependent-care deficit is the core of the general theory because it expresses the human condition that exists when people require nursing. The theory of self-care deficit has conceptual articulations with both the theory of self-care and the theory of nursing system.

The conceptual system represented in Figure 5-1 shows the broad and essential conceptual elements of the three theoretical constructs, as well as the relations among the constructs. The theory of self-care is represented in the figure by the patient element of "self-care"; the theory of self-care deficit by the patient elements of "self-care agency" and "therapeutic self-care demand," and by the represented deficit relationship between agency and demand; and the theory of nursing system by the articulation of the nurse element of "nursing agency," with the patient elements of "self-care agency" and "therapeutic self-care demand" and the relation between them. The activation of nursing agency by nurses to regulate the state of patients' self-care agency and therapeutic self-care demands is nursing. The product of this activation is identified as a nursing system (Nursing Development Conference Group, 1979, p. 107).

BROAD CONCEPTUAL ELEMENTS

The work of development and validation of the six broad, essential or core conceptual elements of the theory extended over the period 1965 to 1971. This work included the investigation of questions, the description and analyses of nursing practice situations, nursing cases, and categories of cases, as well as hypothetical deductive approaches. The work processes are described in some detail in the 1973 and 1979 publications of the Nursing Development Conference Group, in the chapters titled "A General Concept of Nursing" and "Dynamics of Concept Development."

Self-care and dependent care are understood as learned goal-oriented behaviors. As an element in the theory, self-care is understood as a process element involving motion or change produced by individuals in reality situations. From an action and result seeking perspective, self-care is understood as regulating in both human functioning and human development. Regulation is produced by action directed by individuals to themselves (or to their dependents) and to their environments. Self-care actions of individuals produced in some sequential pattern constitute action systems that are referred to as self-care systems. Required regulatory actions are termed self-care requisites; these have been identified and classed as universal, developmental, and health deviation-type requisites (Orem, 1985, pp. 84-100). In reality situations, some discrete self-actions are observable as they are performed. Information about individuals' engagement in self-care can also be elicited through questioning.

Therapeutic self-care demand as a conceptual element in the theory of nursing is an extension of the entities termed self-care requisites, that is, the regulatory actions required by individuals if they are to remain alive, develop, and function, and enjoy human well-being. Therapeutic self-care demand is a humanly constructed entity that summarizes the number and kinds of care measures that need to be performed if identified and particularized self-care requisites of individuals are to be met and the needed regulations of human functioning or development achieved. The calculation of an ideal or an adjusted therapeutic self-care demand requires valid answers to the following questions:

1. What human and environmental factors should be regulated through self-care?

2. Are there factors that interfere with the accomplishment of these regulations?

3. What means or technologies are valid for bringing about each regulation surmounting or overcoming existent interferences?

4. What sets of regulatory care measures must be performed to use selected technologies to attain regulation of functioning or development at some point within an acceptable and attainable range?

The summation of care measures judged necessary to maintain or preserve the life, health, or well-being of individuals constitutes an urgent requirement for action by individuals themselves or when action limitations exist by others (Orem, 1985, pp. 87-89, 100-102).

Self-care agency (dependent care agency) is understood as a complex property or attribute of individuals that enables one to determine requirements for and to take effective action to meet the known, particularized regulatory requisites of individuals. Within the theory of nursing, self-care agency is understood as a summation of the human capabilities needed for performing self-care operations in reality situations. From an action perspective, self-care agency is understood as the human capability to engage in that form of deliberative action named self-care.

Self-care agency and *therapeutic self-care demand* are related or ordered concepts within the structure of the theory of nursing.

The relation involves on the one hand some kind and amount of capability for the action termed self-care and on the other hand some known urgent requirement to engage in such care. The relation between the two conceptual entities may be a relation of equality or inequality. Self-care agency may be equal to the meeting of the therapeutic self-care demand, it may extend beyond the requisite capabilities, or it may be consituted from less than the requisite capabilities. In the latter case, a *self-care deficit* is said to exist. Self-care deficits may be existent, described deficits for current engagement in required self-care, or they may be predicted for occurrence in the future according to projected changes in self-care agency or in the therapeutic self-care demand (Orem, 1985, pp. 105-130; Nursing Development Conference Group, 1973, pp. 181-200).

Nursing agency is understood as a complex property or attribute of nurses developed through specialized education and training in nursing sciences and in the art of nursing. From an action perspective it is a human property that is enabling for nurses to engage in the diagnostic, prescriptive, and regulatory operations necessary to design and produce systems of nursing care for persons with self-care or dependent care deficits associated with the health state or health care requirements of persons in need of care.

Nursing system is understood as a product of nurses' activation of their nursing agency to determine the values of patients' self-care agency and therapeutic self-care demands, to determine and regulate the relations between them, and to ensure that therapeutic self-care demands are met effectively and that action capabilities are protected. Nursing is a dynamic process that produces a system of action, a care system through which patients' actual or potential self-care capabilities are protected, the exercise or development of their self-care agency is regulated, and their therapeutic self-care demands are calculated and continuously met.

This conceptualization of nursing systems is understood as technological, that is, focused on the specific functions of nursing in human society. In reality situations, technological nursing systems are produced within the context of active interpersonal systems that are legitimized by the contractual relations of nurses and patients within the social context of nursing practice situations (Nursing Development Conference Group, 1979, pp. 106-117; Orem, 1985, pp. 148-149).

A PERIPHERAL CONCEPT

The construct of *basic conditioning factors* is understood within the theory as affecting the specific values of the core elements of the theory at various times. Factors include those associated with age, sexual features, developmental state, health state, sociocultural orientation, socioeconomic elements, health care system elements, family system elements, and pattern of living. These factors condition the values of patients' self-care agency and therapeutic self-care demands, as well as the means that are valid for meeting self-care requisites and in regulating self-care agency at particular times in the lives of individuals. Basis conditioning factors are not descriptive or explanatory of the structure of the core concepts of the theory but condition them in various ways (Nursing Development Conference Group, 1979, pp. 169-179). For example, both age and developmental state factors condition the values at which universal self-care requisites should be met as well as the means for meeting them.

The components of the construct, basic conditioning factors, are interrelated and in their relationships have meaning for the quality and quantity of nursing, as well as for other forms of health care required by members of populations. For example, major diagnostic categories and diagnostic related groups (DRGs) used as bases for medical peer review and hospital reimbursement incorporate three basic conditioning factors: health state factors (primary and secondary medical diagnoses and complications), health care system factors (surgery), and age.

Although DRGs are medically oriented, nurses can move to explicate their nursing features if DRGs are viewed as conditioning the characteristics of self-care agency and therapeutic self-care demands.

Theoretical Concepts and the Reality of Nursing Practice Situations

The expression of understandings about any sector of reality is preceded by the formulation of insights as concepts. If one is told that there is a large excavated area in a specific city block and later is told that at this location there is a twelve-story office building with parking facilities, what is said conforms to the two experienced realities. However, theoretical concepts such as self-care agency, therapeutic self-care demand, and nursing agency differ from real concepts such as an excavated area or a twelve-story office building. The substantive structure—the secondary concepts within self-care agency and other concepts of the theory—must be uncovered to reveal entities that can be experienced and observed in the world of the nurse. There are specific methods used to accomplish this process (Nursing Development Conference Group, 1979).

Terms become more specified in meaning with use. For example, the term self-care agency came into consistent use by members of the Nursing Development Conference Group in 1969 to refer to the human capability to engage in self-care. Prior to the formalization of this concept, the terms self-care abilities and limitations were in use as referents for capabilities for self-care. The substantive structure of self-care agency is now understood by nurses who use the self-care deficit theory of nursing as being constituted from three distinct but related types of human capabilities, human properties or traits, that are enabling for engagement in self-care. These are identified as follows:

1. Capabilities to perform three types of self-care operations, namely, estimative, decision making, and productive self-care operations. For example, a person at home experiences a change in cardiac functioning and identifies, on the basis of current and past experiences, the condition of auricular fibrillation. The person examines the options that are open, for example, to go about regular activities with or without modification, to take a prescribed medication, to consult the physician, or to continue to monitor vital signs. This person has knowledge of things about which judgments and decisions must be made. The person is acquiring information and making judgments about what is and what can and should be done, makes a decision about what will be done, and then engages in actions specified by the decision.

2. Ten enabling capabilities known as the power components

of self-care agency. These empowering capabilities must be developed and operational in order for individuals to perform one or all of the identified types of self-care operations in reality situations. An example of a power component is the controlled use of available physical energy that is sufficient for the initiation and continuation of self-care operations.

3. Five sets of foundational capabilities and dispositions including two sets of basic capabilities necessary for any form of deliberate action, one set of knowing and doing capabilities, one set of dispositions affecting goals sought, and a set of significant orientative capabilities and dispositions. These sets were developed (Backscheider, NDCG, 1979) as a survey list of general capabilities requisite for engagement in self-care. They include, for example, sensation, perception, memory, operational knowing, and health orientation (Backscheider, NDCG, 1979).

It is evident that these components of the substantive structure of self-care agency point to entities in concrete nursing practice situations about which information can be obtained.

The specific entities within any one of the three named types of human capabilities or human features can be utilized in the investigation of real situations of nursing practice for purposes of nursing practice or nursing research. An example is Backscheider's (Nursing Development Conference Group, 1979, pp. 184-231) study of operational knowing in members of an adult, ambulatory clinic population, some members of which were educationally deprived. During the initial period of operation of a nursing clinic there was evidence that some persons did not acquire or use new knowledge toward the goal of regulating their diabetic condition. In the role of nonparticipant observer during instructional sessions, Backscheider made behavioral observations of exchanges between the clinic nurse and the patients, noting the features of patients' verbalizations.

Observations were made from live and recorded exchanges between patients and the clinic nurse (Nursing Development Conference Group, 1979, pp. 184-231). Observations yielded data about seven modes of operational knowing. Findings led to the conclusion that some members of the clinic population on the basis of inferences about their operations of thought did not conform to those associated with reasoning on propositional verbal statements. Two groups were identified from the members of the clinic population: those whose inferred operations of thought were experience oriented with a focus on the here and now, and those whose inferred mental operations were focused on concrete or experienced wholes with some understanding of relationships and boundaries. Modes of operational knowing were described for each group and six identifying characteristics were expressed for each group.

The described investigation provided results that were helpful to nurses in the immediate provision of nursing to members of the clinic population. It also provides a basis for developing research methodologies for investigations of operational knowing that are important for nurses and nursing. It is an example of the use of a human development model in the search for understanding of one feature of the complex human capability named self-care agency (Nursing Development Conference Group, 1979, pp. 184-231).

Stages of Development of a General Theory of Nursing

Understanding nursing with formalization of the domain and boundaries of nursing as a practical science is viewed as a developmental process. The works of other nurses as well as those of this writer, suggest five stages in the development of a general theory of nursing. A stage is understood in terms of the occurrence of insights or sets of insights about the essential features of nursing. It is what the insights are about, the kinds of data or images, that provides the bases for distinguishing and naming stages of development. Stages should be understood as interlocking and overlapping. The stage development of the general theory of nursing was formalized in early 1985.

The five stages of development are identified in Figure 5-3 and are briefly described here.

1. The stage of describing and explaining nursing. The product of this state is the formulated and expressed self-care deficit theory of nursing and its conceptual system.

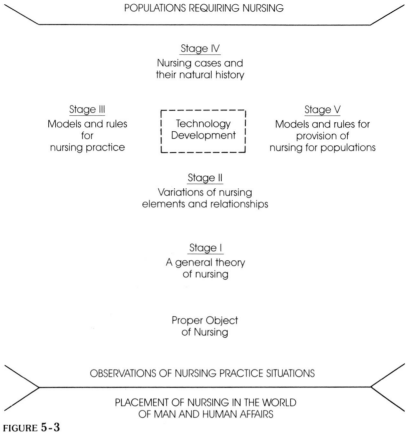

FIGURE 5-3
Stages of understanding nursing.

2. The stage of describing and explaining the range of variation of the broad conceptual elements of the theory, as well as the range of variation in their substantive conceptual components. Results in this stage include, for example, variations in self-care agency along the dimensions of development, operability, and adequacy as well as variations in *operational knowing* described in the prior section. *Therapeutic self-care demand* can vary along dimensions of components, stability, and complexity.

3. The stage of formulating models and rules of nursing practice with determination of the validity and reliability of models under some mix and range of conditions and circumstances.

4. The stage of describing and classifying nursing cases, the ranges of variation of their distinguishing features, and their natural history.

5. The stage of formulating models and rules for providing nursing for populations. Such models are nursing product design models essential for use in organized nursing services.

As shown in Figure 5-3, the formulation of technologies and the establishment of their validity and reliability should proceed during all five stages.

Some combination of the five stages may be in process at the same time and each stage can be understood in terms of its phases of development. For example, Figure 5-2 represents an early phase of stage 1, the stage of describing and explaining nursing. In Figure 5-2, nurse is related to patient, types of self-care are identified but not named, and basic conditioning factors are distributed around the patient. Figure 5-1 is the result of a later phase of development in stage 1.

Present Status of Stage Development

Stage 1 has been brought to a high degree of maturity but continues under development. Stage 2 continues in process. The work of development of the substantive structure of self-care agency, and the study of its specific elements in reality situations is an example of stage 2 development.

Stages 3, 4, and 5 have nurses taking the stance of nursing practitioners in relation to persons requiring nursing. In Stage 3 development, practice models and rules can be formulated at varying levels of generality or specificity. Nursing practice rules are related to the contractual, interpersonal, and technological features of nursing practice (Orem, 1985, pp. 240-244).

Models of nursing practice can be primarily structural or primarily process models, or a combination of the two. For example, wholly compensatory, partly compensatory, and supportive educative nursing system models are primarily structural models because they specify the nurse role and that patient role based on valid methods of helping in light of qualitative and quantitative characteristics of patients' self-care agency (Orem, 1985, pp. 151-154).

The procedural models of the Horn and Swain study (1977) are process models for determining: (1) whether universal and selected health deviation self-care requisites are being met; and (2) the adequacy of knowledge, skill development, and performance capabilities for meeting particularized self-care requisites. Rauckhorst's models of nursing system variables in the stages of cerebrovascular accidents, while primarily structural in form, have process implications (Nursing Development Conference Group, 1979, pp. 256-272).

The work of Underwood (n.d.) and the nurses who follow her design for nursing for persons with chronic mental illness has produced a process model with structural foundations. Methods of helping are specified in relation to manifestations of patient capabilities for action with specification of nurse and patient roles in meeting self-care requisites.

Backscheider's work related to operational knowing when validated (as cited in Nursing Development Conference Group, 1979, pp. 184-231) could be developed into practice models for nursing individuals who may have special difficulty with the estimative, or the judgment and decision making, or the production operations of self-care. This work also has implications for the development of a diagnostic technology.

Preliminary work is underway toward development of practice models for nursing for multiperson units such as families and residence groups (Orem, 1984, pp 43-47; 1985, pp, 251-255).

Stage 4, the stage of describing the classfying nursing cases, focuses on concrete instances of persons under the care of nurses who are able to describe: (1) characterizing nursing relevant features of these persons and the history of their development, (2) actions of nurses and patients, and (3) discernible results of these actions. This stage yields similarities and dissimilarities in nursing cases for the variables self-care agency, therapeutic self-care demand, and nursing agency, and also information about range of effectiveness of diagnostic and regulatory techniques and technologies. The stage also yields the kind and amount of evidence necessary for making valid nursing judgments and decisions when specific combinations of conditions prevail.

Stage 4 developments can be made by nursing practitioners who are keen observers with practical insight, who recognize questions for investigation and questions for reflection, and who are aware of and understand the relationship between what they know and what they do. Such nursing practitioners accurately document what occurs and what is done, keep records, and study them for the purpose of improving their practice and for adding to the practical science of nursing. Some nursing practitioners are presently engaged in describing nursing cases within the framework of the self-care deficit theory of nursing.

Stage 5, the stage of formulating models and rules for providing nursing to populations, has a dual focus. Developments in this stage result in descriptions of populations in need of nursing and in models and rules for providing nursing to each population or subpopulation. Population is a class concept. The class is constituted from individual members of the population. For example, the whole number of people in a community or a geographic area is a population. Individual members of the class can form smaller units according to modes of organization of units that are selected because they are capable of being interpreted as to apply to the actual world. Subclasses can be combined, as for example, unimmunized preschool children.

Hospital populations can be described in terms of basic conditioning factors that can be judged as actively affecting the values of self-care agency and therapeutic self-care demand of members of the hospital population. Inferences can then be made about requisite values of the nursing agency of legitimate nurses.

Development of models and rules for the provision of nursing for populations requires data to describe populations in need of nursing by classes and subclasses including combinations thereof as well as the duration of their requirements for nursing. Model development also requires that nurses use the hypothetical deductive method in the identification of requirements for nursing for each of the identified classes and subclasses of a population. (Nursing Development Conference Group, 1979, pp. 249-284).

Functions of a General
Theory of Nursing

The self-care deficit theory of nursing and its conceptual elements in their relationships provide a way for nurses to understand that sector of reality which constitutes the world of the nurse. The theory should not be viewed and used as an ideology, as when everything perceived in nursing practice situations is viewed as fitting within the theory. The general theory indicates the proper object of nursing, the elements within nursing's domain, and the boundaries of nursing, as well as the end product of nursing and the human results sought through nursing.

This general theory of nursing and its conceptual structure with the products of its five developmental stages are viewed as parts of nursing science. Nursing sciences are accepted as one of seven disciplines of knowledge that focus on nurses and nursing. The other identified disciplines include nursing's social field, nursing as a profession and occupation, nursing jurisprudence, nursing history, nursing ethics, and nursing economics (Orem, 1985, p. 77). Content from all seven fields are included in nursing courses in programs of education preparatory for entry to nursing practice. Nursing science is critical for inclusion in such programs.

Nurses can move more effectively to develop nursing sciences if they have a clear view of their form and structure. A clear view is not easy to attain. The self-care deficit theory of nursing in its five developmental stages aids in attaining such a view. The theory specifies both theoretical and practical components of nursing science. Theoretical components point to articulation of nursing elements with concepts, facts and points of theory from other disciplines. The areas of articulation indicate foci for development of applied nursing science (Orem, 1985, pp. 39-46).

APPENDIX A
Explanatory Terms: The Self-Care Deficit Theory of Nursing

SET 1. PATIENT-ORIENTED TERMS

Legitimate patients of nurses are persons whose therapeutic self-care demands exceed their self-care agency due to some combination of health or health-related factors.

Self-care is a learned activity: it is behavior; it exists in reality situations. It is action directed by individuals to themselves or their environments in order to regulate their own functioning and development in the interests of life, integrated functioning, and well-being.

Dependent care is care as described above directed by responsible adults to socially dependent individuals, children or adults.

Therapeutic self-care demand is a summation of the measures of care required at moments in time in order for individuals to meet existent regulatory action requirements (self-care requisites) to maintain life or to maintain or promote integrated functioning and general well-being.

Self-care agency is the complex capability of individuals for *determining* their therapeutic self-care demands and for *producing* care specified by an ideal or adjusted therapeutic self-care demand. Self-care agency may be operative outside of or within systems of nursing care.

Dependent-care agency is the capability to engage in these operations for a dependent person.

SET 2. NURSE AND NURSING-ORIENTED TERMS

Legitimate nurses are persons who have the sets of qualities or characteristics symbolized by the term nursing agency.

Nursing agency (when activated) is enabling for nurses

1. To engage in operations to establish the legitimacy of others as patients of nurses.

2. To engage in operations to judge the adequacy of their own

nursing agency and that of other nurses in specific nursing practice situations.

3. To perform diagnostic operations to identify
   a. Existent, emerging, and projected self-care requisites including their regulatory functions and the values at which they should be met
   b. Developed and operational self-care capabilities
   c. The presence, the nature of, and the action limiting effects of conditions and circumstances that interfere with engagement in self-care

4. To establish the adequacy or inadequacy of the self-care agency of individuals in relation to meeting their therapeutic self-care demands

5. To prescribe therapeutic self-care demands for individuals and patients' roles and nurses' roles in meeting patients' therapeutic self-care demands and in regulating the exercise or development of patients' self-care agency

6. To engage in productive operations to bring about combinations of the following nursing results that can accrue over time
   a. The therapeutic self-care demand: (1) describes factors in patients or their environments that must be held steady within a range or brought within and held within a range of values over which factors can vary, (2) particularizes the values at which requisites should be met, (3) identifies methods or technologies for meeting particularized requisites, and (4) identifies and organizes the sets of actions to be performed to use selected technologies in meeting particularized requisites
   b. The human bases for self-care agency are protected and the therapeutic self-care demand is met
   c. Self-care agency is or is becoming equal to estimating and meeting the therapeutic self-care demand
   d. Self-care agency is exercised to produce a system of self-care that is effective in meeting constituent parts or the totality of the therapeutic self-care demand

Nursing systems are action systems that are produced as nurses engage in the foregoing operations of nursing practice relating themselves to patients and at times to members of patients' families through their selection and use of one or a combination of ways of helping, namely, acting for or doing for another, guiding another, supporting another, providing a developmental environment, teaching another. The operations of nursing practice conjoined with ways of helping are performed in order to determine and meet patients' therapeutic self-care demands and to regulate the exercise or development of patients' self-care agency. Such technological nursing systems are dependent upon the existence of interpersonal systems that result from contact and association of individuals that make possible interaction. Interpersonal systems between legitimate patients of nurses and legitimate nurses develop within contractual relationships which articulate with the encompassing social system.

Sources: Orem, 1985, pp. 24-27, 132-172, 209-247; and Nursing Development Conference Group, 1979, pp. 105-127.

REFERENCES

Horn, B. J., and Swain, M. A. (1977). *Development of criterion measures of nursing care*, Vol. 1. Springfield, VA: University of Michigan and National Center for Health Services Research, National Technical Information Service, pub. no. 267-004.

Lonergan, B. J. F. (1958). Insight, A study of human understanding. New York: Philosophical Library.

Nursing Development Conference Group (1979). Concept formalization of nursing: process and product, 2nd ed. Boston: Little, Brown & Co.

Orem, D. E. (1959). *Guides for developing curricula for the education of practical nurses*. Washington, D. C.: U. S. Department of Health, Education and Welfare, Office of Education.

Orem, D. E., ed. (1979). Nursing Development Conference Group: Concept formalization in nursing: Process and product, 2nd ed. Boston: Little, Brown & Co.

Orem, D. E. (1984). "Orem's conceptual model and community health nursing." *In* M. K. Asay and C. C. Ossler, eds., *Conceptual models of nursing, application in community health nursing*. Chapel Hill, NC: Department of Public Health Nursing, School of Public Health, University of North Carolina at Chapel Hill.

Orem, D. E. (1985). *Nursing: Concepts of practice*, 3rd ed. New York: McGraw-Hill Book Co.

Underwood, P. R. (n. d.). *Tools for implementation of self-care deficit theory*, Vol. 1. San Francisco: School of Nursing, Department of Mental Health and Community Nursing, University of California, San Francisco.

Wallace, W. A. (1979). *From a realist point of view: Essays in the philosophy of science*. Essay 13: "Being scientific in a practice discipline." Washington, D. C.: University Press of America.

A Critique of Orem's Theory

MARY JANE SMITH

This chapter presents a critique of Orem's general theory of nursing as presented in her latest work, the third edition of *Nursing Concepts of Practice*. The following discussion focuses on the assumptions, concepts, and propositions—the essential elements of a theory—rather than relating the specific detail in the work.

Structure

HISTORICAL EVOLUTION

Orem is a pioneer in the work toward the conceptualization of the object of nursing. She has stated that her "interest about the domain and boundaries of nursing was piqued during the 1950's"

91

(Orem, 1985, p. 18). A beginning formalization of the domain and boundaries of nursing was expressed in 1956 and refined in 1959. (Orem, 1985, p. 18). In 1958 and 1959 she participated in a project to upgrade vocational nurse training that sought to explicate the nursing component of vocational nursing. Orem's insight into the human condition and the requirements for nursing led her to formulate the following idea:

The inability of a person to provide continuously for self the amount and quality of required self-care because of the situation of personal health is the object of nursing.

This formulation led her to the idea of self-care, which she published in 1959 as *Guides for the Developing Curriculum for the Education of Practical Nurses.* Orem's *Nursing: Concepts of Practice* was first published in 1971 and is now in its third edition (1985). Refinement of her work was also published in 1973 and 1979 under the title *Concept Formalization in Nursing: Process and Product.*

PHILOSOPHICAL ASSUMPTIONS

Orem characterizes five assumptions that underlie the general theory of nursing (Orem, 1985, pp. 33-34):

1. Human beings require continuous deliberate inputs to themselves and their environments in order to remain alive and function in accord with natural human endowments.

2. Human agency, the power to act deliberately, is exercised in the form of care of self and others in identifying needs for and in making needed inputs.

3. Mature human beings experience privations in the form of limitations for action in care of self and others involving the making of life-sustaining and function-regulating inputs.

4. Human agency is exercised in discovering, developing, and transmitting to others ways and means to identify needs for and make inputs to self and others.

5. Groups of human beings with structured relationships cluster tasks and allocate responsibilities for providing care to group
members who experience privations for making required deliberate input to self and others.

These assumptions refer to human beings and human agency.
The first assumption is a belief about the requirement of human
beings to remain alive and to function naturally. The requirement
is for continuous, deliberate input to self and to the environment.
The third assumption, also about mature human beings, refers to
the experience of privations for actions in care of self and others.
The actions involve the making of life-sustaining and function-regulating input. Mature human beings experience limitations in the
making of life-sustaining and function-regulating inputs. The fifth
belief is about groups of human beings, and seems to be a synthesis
of the first and third assumptions. Groups of human beings allocate
tasks and responsibilities for providing care to members who experience privations for making required deliberate input to self and
others. The second assumption refers to human agency as the
power to act deliberately by caring for self and others, which involves identifying and making needed inputs. The fourth assumption also about human agency, is the power to act deliberately and
transmit to others ways and means for identifying needs and making inputs to self and others. These assumptions are about human
beings acting deliberately, identifying needs, caring for self and others, experiencing privations, and obtaining life-sustaining and function-regulating inputs.

Orem's five assumptions, although stated explicitly, do not express a singular belief in a clear way at either the philosophical or
more general level of discourse. In the logical progression of theory
development, the philosophical precedes the conceptual, which
precedes the empirical. Thus, Orem's assumptions should be written at a higher, more general level of discourse.

The assumptions refer to the concrete, namely, acting deliberately, identifying needs, caring for self and others, experiencing
deprivations, and obtaining life-sustaining and function-regulating
inputs. When theory development begins at the empirical level, the
logical progression downward to the proposition statement is trun-
cated and becomes circular; the assumptions set the pattern of

abstraction and the range of facts that the theory fits. Stating assumptions at the concrete level of discourse limits the theory by restricting movement up and down the ladder of discourse. A theory is supposed to guide practice and research as well as provide a spin-off point for the generation of new knowledge. But the language used in Orem's assumptions restricts the usefulness of the theory.

PRINCIPLES, CONCEPTS, AND PROPOSITIONS

There are no stated principles in Orem's work, although there are concepts and propositions. The six concepts therein are self-care, therapeutic self-care demand, self-care agency, self-care deficit, nursing agency, and nursing system. There are three theories that comprise what Orem calls the general theory of nursing. These theories are related to self-care deficit, self-care, and nursing system. Each is expressed in a set of propositions and presuppositions.

DEFINITION OF MAN

Human beings are the main referents in the assumptions of the general history. These assumptions have already been addressed. An elaboration of human beings is found in Orem's Chapter 8 (1985, p. 174): Human beings are distinguishable from other living things by their capacity (1) to reflect upon themselves and the environment; (2) to symbolize what they experience; and (3) to use symbolic creations (ideas and words) in thinking and communicating and in guiding efforts to do and make things that are beneficial to themselves and others.

A human being is a unity that can be viewed as functioning biologically, symbolically, and socially. Human beings are posited as a substantial or real unity whose parts are formed and attain perfection through the differentiation of the whole during processes of development (Orem, 1985).

DEFINITION OF HEALTH

In Orem's examination of health and nursing (1985, pp. 173-197), concepts discussed include health, health as state, positions about health and well-being, nursing and health care, the nursing focus versus the medical focus, primary, secondary and tertiary levels of prevention, classification of nursing systems on health focus, variations in health care, and health care systems. Health is viewed as a term to describe living things when they are structurally and functionally whole or sound. Health is the state of wholeness or integrity of human beings. Any deviation from normal structure or functioning is referred to as "an absence of health" (p. 174). Health state refers to a set of determined values of specified human characteristics that simultaneously reveal some aspects of the person's existence. The specified characteristics when taken together as a set describe the state of the person at a particular time. Health and well-being refer to two different states. Health is characterized by soundness or wholeness of developed human structures and of bodily and mental functioning. Well-being refers to a person's perceived condition of existence, and as a state is characterized by experiences of contentment, pleasure, happiness, spiritual experiences, movement toward fulfillment of one's self ideal and continued personalization.

RELATIONSHIP BETWEEN MAN AND HEALTH

Orem (1985) relates person and health first as a state of integrity or wholeness that can be evaluated on the basis of feeling well or sick (p. 173). This evaluation implies that individuals know what health means to them. Second, health is "that which makes a person human (form of mental life), operating in conjunction with physiological and psychological mechanisms and a material structure (biological life) and in relation to coexistence with other human beings (interpersonal and social life)" (p. 174). The physical, psychological, interpersonal, and social aspects of health are inseparable in the individual. And third, health is related to "human beings" as persons and the structural-functional differentiations of human beings (p. 180).

The views about Man and health described in Orem's chapter eight are presented at the philosophical level. It is regrettable that these views are not explicated in the assumptions of the general theory of nursing and that these assumptions are not reflected in the definitions of the concepts.

Process

CORRESPONDENCE

Established Knowledge of Man and Health

The test of correspondence comes with analyzing how the theory relates to established knowledge. Orem's theory is rooted in the work of Henderson (1955). There is little evidence of rooting the concepts and propositions in explicit theoretical literature, yet this is understandable, since the explication of the assumptions, concepts, and propositions is rooted in Orem's early experience in nursing. Her theory contains traditional commonly held views of what nurses do in the service to people. While the theory is not a medical model, it does correspond well with medicine. Indeed the nursing focus takes into account the medical point of view as well as the patient's point of view (Orem, 1985, p. 185). This correspondence with medicine reaffirms nursing in its traditional role.

The focus of the general theory of nursing is the self-care deficit theory. The deficit relationship is a determination of the limitations that render a person "incapable of continuous self-care" (p. 34). The emphasis on the "deficit relationship where care abilities are less than those required for meeting a known self-care demand" (p. 35) leads to a focus on disorder. The focus on disorder emphasizes the negative and restricts the potential of nursing to society. Ellis believes that nursing in the movement to a unique science must be directed from a focus on human capacities and strength (Ellis, 1982, p. 409). Orem's focus on the deficit relationship as to the core of the theory leads away from human strengths and capacities.

Interrelation of Concepts at Same Level of Discourse

The clarity in Orem's assumptions, concepts, and propositions is obfuscated by her rigid adherence to the empirical level of discourse from her assumptions through her propositions. Meaning is not clarified by the definitions. Circularity arises in Orem's attempt to add substance by expanding verbosity. There is a pattern of excessive verbosity in describing the empirical and circularity obfuscating meaning. The effort to explain the meaning of a term by adding more concrete terms only makes the obvious more complex.

Relationship to Paradigmatic Perspectives and Philosophical Assumptions

Orem's general theory of nursing fits with the totality paradigm of nursing. In the totality paradigm, Man is considered a bio-psycho-social spiritual being who reacts and adapts to the environment. Man is an organism whose behavior can be measured and predicted as well as changed through management of the environment. Health is considered a state of well-being that can be identified and altered by health professionals according to social expectations (Parse and others, 1985).

Description and Meaning of Principles, Concepts, and Propositions

Concepts. Though there are no principles posited, six concepts are identified in Orem's theory: self-care, therapeutic self-care demand, self-care agency, self-care deficit, nursing agency, and nursing system (Orem, 1985, p. 31). Self-care is defined as "the production of actions directed to self or to the environment in order to regulate one's functioning and well-being" (p. 31). This means, then, that self-care is self-action to regulate integrated functioning and well-being. Therapeutic self-care demand is defined as "the measures of care required at moments in time in order to meet

existent requisites for regulatory action to maintain life and to maintain or promote health and development and general well being"
(p. 31). The meaning of this concept is not clear. Therapeutic is
generally defined as relating to the treatment of disease or disorder
by remedial agents and demand refers to asking and requesting. It
is expected that the definitions of theoretical concepts agree with
the general language definitions of the terms.

Self-care agency is defined as "the complex capability for action that is activated in the performance of the actions or operations
of self care" (p. 31). This refers to capability to act in the care of
self or others. How is self-care agency different from self-care when
self-care is defined as the production of actions? If actions are produced, then one is capable of producing. They are very close in
definition. Self-care deficit is defined as "a relationship between
self-care agency and therapeutic self-care demand in which self-
care agency is not adequate to meet the known therapeutic self-
care demand" (p. 31). This refers to an inability to care for self
which is related to demands exceeding actions. These four concepts are tied very closely to each other by definition. It could be
questioned whether there are four concepts, or whether there is
one concept of self-care with points of elaboration (capability, demand, and deficit) on aspects of self-care.

Nursing agency, the fifth concept, is defined as "the complex
capability for action that is activated by nurses in their determination of needs for design of and production of nursing for persons
with a range of types of self-care deficits" (p. 31). This concept
refers to determining the needs of, and designing and providing
nursing for, persons with self-care deficits. Nursing system, the sixth
concept, which is closely tied to nursing agency, is defined as "a
continuing series of actions produced when nurses link one way or
a number of ways of helping to their own actions or the actions of
persons under care that are directed to meet those persons self-
care demands or to regulate their self-care agency" (p. 31). The
meaning of this concept is not clear. It entails groups of nurses
engaging in nursing agency to meet therapeutic self-care demands.
Since nursing system includes nursing agency, it could be concluded that the concept is nursing system. It could also be concluded that there are only two concepts (self-care and nursing
system) to the theory.

The six concepts of the theory are defined at a concrete level of abstraction, yet Orem states that "the concepts are theoretical and do not relate to specific observable conditions" (p. 31). On close examination, it is clear that the concepts as defined are very focused and at the empirical level of discourse. The purpose of explicit definition is to clarify, simplify, and systematize concepts (Kaplan, 1964, p. 271). Orem's definitions fall short of this requirement.

It is a further expectation of definitions that the definition not include the term or part of the term to be defined. Yet self-care is defined as the production of actions directed to self; therapeutic self-care demand is defined as the measures of care; the definition of self-care agency includes self-care; the definition of self-care deficit includes the term self-care (three times); and the definition of nursing agency and nursing system both include the term nurse. This circularity limits interpretation and substance. When the term is used to define itself, the term turns right back on itself rather than being expanded in meaning.

Propositions. The six concepts related to self-care, therapeutic self-care demand, self-care deficit, self-care agency, nursing agency, and nursing system are further explicated as the three theories related to the general theory. Each of the three theories is expressed in a set of propositions and presuppositions. Orem defines the theory of self-care deficit or dependent care deficit as constituting the "core of the general theory of nursing" (Orem, 1985, p. 34). In fact, Orem wrote that "the general theory of nursing is referred to as the self-care deficit theory of nursing" (p. 38). The self-care deficit theory includes six propositions and two sets of presuppositions.

A proposition of a theory is a statement that relates two or more foundational concepts in a way that guides practice and research. One would expect that the six concepts listed above are related or tied together in the propositions of the self-care deficit theory. The first proposition states that "persons who take action to provide their own self-care or care for dependents have specialized capabilities for action (p. 25). This proposition is a further elaboration of self-care agency. The second proposition states that "the individual's abilities to engage in self-care or dependent care

are conditioned by age, developmental state, life experience, sociocultural orientation, health, and available resources" (p. 35). This proposition introduces dependent care, which is not mentioned in the six concepts and seems to be more of a statement of belief about conditions relative to self-care. The third proposition states that "the relationship of individuals' abilities for self-care or dependent care to the qualitative and quantitative self-care or dependent-care demand can be determined when the value of each is known" (p. 35). This proposition relates the concepts of self-care and therapeutic self-care demand in a rather simplistic way. It is like saying that when the values for A and B are known, the A-B relationship can be determined. The fourth proposition states that "the relationship between care abilities and care demand can be defined in terms of equal to, less than, more than" (p. 35). This is a further elaboration on the concept of self-care deficit and is thus a definition. The fifth proposition states that "nursing is a legitimate service when: (a) Care abilities are less than those required for meeting a known self-care demand (a deficit relationship); (b) Self-care or dependent-care abilities exceed or are equal to those required for meeting the current self-care demand but a future deficit relationship can be foreseen because of predictable decreases in care abilities, qualitative or quantitative increases in the care demand, or both" (p. 35). It defines legitimate nursing through the concept of self-care deficit and therefore seems to be a statement of belief. The sixth proposition states that "persons with existing or projected care deficits are in, or can expect to be in, states of social dependency that legitimate a nursing relationship" (p. 35). It would seem that the third and sixth propositions do not interrelate the basic concepts in a meaningful way.

Orem also describes presuppositions after each set of propositions. A presupposition is generally defined as something that comes before. There seems to be a logical incongruence then, in stating the presupposition after the supposition. The presuppositions in set one are further elaborations on self-care; those in set two, general statements of belief. The inclusion of both tends to obfuscate rather than clarify understanding of the self-care deficit theory.

This is an example of an analysis of one of Orem's theories of nursing. It is the core theory on which the other two are modeled.

There is a pattern in the structure of the propositions whereby the basic concepts are not related and the presence of very generally stated presuppositions serve to lead the reader away from the central notion of the theory. This is true for all three of Orem's theories.

COHERENCE

Relation of Theory to Other Theories

The general theory of self-care is unique. It does not specifically relate to other theories or frameworks in or out of the discipline of nursing. It does have some common beliefs with other frameworks that connect it to the totality paradigm, as pointed out above.

Logical Flow from Assumptions to Propositions

There is a problem with the logical flow of the theory from assumptions through propositions. The logical problem stems from the absence of discrete levels of discourse within the theory. The theory does not provide the intellectual impetus for movement up and down the ladder of abstraction; thus a circulatory pattern ensues in the quest to advance knowledge.

Symmetry and Aesthetics

Augros and Stanciu (1984) have set forth the idea that beauty is the primary standard of truth. There are three elements of scientific beauty: simplicity, which includes completeness and economy; harmony, which includes symmetry; and brilliance, which includes clarity. While aesthetics is a valid criterion of a theory, not all theorists attend to this with the same amount of rigor. And one must keep in mind that beauty is in the eye of the beholder. In summary, Orem's theory is not parsimonious, lacks symmetry, makes the simple complex, and obfuscates clarity.

PRAGMATICS

Use of Theory in Practice and Research

Pragmatics refers to the use of the theory in education, practice, and research. Orem's theory is one of the most widely accepted and used theories in nursing. Fawcett (1984, pp. 196-197) has documented publications citing the use of Orem's theory in practice settings, particularly disease conditions with persons who have a terminal illness, and with children, adolescents, and aged persons. Seventeen references are cited that relate to use of the theory in practice settings (p. 197). Furthermore, the theory has been used as a framework for guiding practice in a variety of health care agencies (p. 197).

The theory also has a wide use as a curriculum framework. It is used in diploma, associate and baccalaureate degree programs. Fawcett has reported that the following baccalaureate programs have used the theory: Georgetown University, University of Southern Mississippi, and the University of Missouri at Columbia (pp. 197-198).

A review of the 1984 issues of *Nursing Research* and *Research in Nursing and Health* has revealed two reported studies on self-care. A study by Hubbard and others (1984), entitled "The Relationship Between Social Support and Self-Care Practices," was published in *Nursing Research*. The study explored what people do to promote healthy life-styles and how they perceive their level of support. Self-care was measured through an instrument that considered nutrition, exercise, relaxation, safety, substance use, and prevention practices. Findings revealed that social support accounted for 34 percent of the variance found in positive health practices. Orem was not cited anywhere in the conceptualization or interpretation of this study on self-care. This study presents an example of the many different views of self-care in the literature today. Johns has written that "despite a widespread interest, there are substantial differences of opinion regarding self-care's definition, its potential as a means of health care delivery, its prioritized research needs and its future role in health care" (Johns, 1985, p. 156).

The second study reported by Dodd (1984) in *Research in*

Nursing and Health, was titled "Measuring Informational Implementation for Chemotherapy Knowledge and Self-Care Behavior." It selected types of information (drug information, side-effect management techniques, or a combination of the two) that nurses could systematically present to cancer patients receiving chemotherapy, and to assess whether the information influences the patient's chemotherapy knowledge, self-care behavior, and general affective state. Self-care was measured using a self-care behavior questionnaire. A self-care behavior performance score was obtained. The hypothesis that side-effects management techniques would increase self-care behaviors was supported at the .01 level of significance. This study was conceptualized using Orem's concept of self-care agency. Dodd found that there was support for Orem's belief that self-care behaviors may be reinforced and augmented by health professionals and that self-care behaviors can be learned.

It must be questioned how a theory with weaknesses in structure, correspondence and coherence can be so strong in pragmatics? Meleis (1985, p.291) has written that the wide acceptance of Orem's work is related to the perspective and language of her theory. Further elaborating, she found that the language of the theory reveals the traditional nursing practice based on human needs and function, thus providing a gentle transition in the shift away from the medical model. The theory incorporates the medical perspective rather than rejects it, and it uses medical language with which most nurses are familiar. Most nurses find a level of comfort in the concrete familiar alignment with the medical model.

Contribution to Nursing Science

Orem has contributed to the evolution of nursing science through the conceptualization and publication of a work that elaborates on the concepts of self-care and nursing action. These have provided a foundation for traditional nursing. This critique of Orem's theory, based on her most recent work, demonstrates difficulties with complete reliance on the empirical level of discourse in the theory; there is obfuscation, circularity of meaning, weak supporting theoretical substance, and logical inadequacy. The assumptions, concepts, and theoretical propositions of Orem's theory were derived as empirically generated theory. An empirically generated theory begins at the concrete level and rises up the ladder of discourse. The transition to the theoretical level requires a rigorous leap upward, the semantics of which reflect a synthesis languaged in the abstract. Orem's theory is rooted and expressed in the empirical. The rigorous leap and the logical presentation of the theoretical level is missing. These difficulties with Orem's work are also documented in the works of Fawcett (1984), Melynk (1983), and Meleis (1985). Orem's theory is strong, however, in documented evidence on its use in education, practice, and research. Her work has created opportunities for scholars to examine the various aspects in the development of nursing science. Because of examinations and discussions such as this, nursing is becoming more specified as a science. This theory has been critiqued in many works and is the curricular framework for many schools of nursing. Orem is indeed a pioneer and is highly respected in nursing for her contributions. She has had the courage to make her ideas public so that they could be critically evaluated in an effort to advance the science of nursing.

REFERENCES

Augros, R. M., and Stanciu, G. N. (1984). *The new story of science*. Bluff, IL.: Regnery Gateway.

Dodd, M. J. (1984). Measuring informational intervention for chemotherapy knowledge and self-care behavior. *Research in Nursing and Health*, 7:43-50.

Ellis, R. (1982). Conceptual issues in nursing. *Nursing Outlook, 30*:406-410.

Fawcett, J. (1984). *Analysis and evaluation of conceptual models of nursing*. Philadelphia: F. A. Davis Co.

Henderson, V. (1955). The nature of nursing. Reprinted in M. E. Meyers, ed., *Nursing Fundamentals*. Dubuque, IA: William. C. Brown Co.

Hubbard, P., Muhlenkamp, A. F. and Brown, N. (1984). The relationship between social support and self-care practices. *Nursing Research, 33*:266-269.

Johns, J. L. (1985). Self-care today: In search of an identity. *Nursing and Health Care, 3*:153-156.

Kaplan, A. (1964), *The conduct of inquiry*. Scranton, PA: Chandler Publishing Co.

Meleis, A. I. (1985). *Theoretical nursing: Development and progress*. Philadelphia: J. B. Lippincott Co.

Melynk, K. A. M. (1983). The process of theory analysis: An examination of the nursing theory of Dorothea E. Orem. *Nursing Research*, *32*:170-174.

Orem, D. E. (1959). *Guides for developing curriculum for the education of practical nurses*. Vocational Division No. 274, Trade and Industrial Education No. 68. Washington, DC: U. S. Department of Health, Education and Welfare.

Orem, D. E. (1985). *Nursing concepts of practice*. New York: McGraw-Hill Book Co.

Parse, R. R., Coyne, A. B., and Smith, M. J. (1985). *Nursing Research: Qualitative methods*. Bowie, MD: Brady Communications.

7

King's Theory of Goal Attainment

IMOGENE M. KING

EDITORIAL PERSPECTIVE

King (1981) describes Man as a rational, sentient, reacting, social, controlling, purposeful, time-oriented, action-oriented organism. The language in this description is consistent with the totality paradigm. Also consistent with this paradigm, King defines health as a dynamic state of well-being. King in a departure from Roy and Orem, specifies an interactional relationship between nurse and client as the basis for her theory. The language of her theory is not from medical science nor is it related to Man's self-care capabilities, but rather it proposes goal attainment as a central factor.

In the following pages, King (1981) sets forth her theory of goal attainment and defines the concepts within this theory. Her beliefs about Man and health surface as grounding for the theory.

Philosophical Assumptions

It is important when setting forth a theory to explain the terminology clearly so that the elements of theory construction can readily be identified (Adams, 1985; Reynolds, 1971).

The philosophical assumptions underlying the theory of goal attainment have been identified and made explicit. Since the focus of the theory (King, 1981, p. 143) is human beings interacting with the environment (which in nursing is with nurses and other health professionals), assumptions about human beings are:

Individuals are social beings.
Individuals are sentient beings.
Individuals are rational beings.
Individuals are reacting beings.
Individuals are perceiving beings.
Individuals are controlling beings.
Individuals are action-oriented beings.
Individuals are time-oriented beings.

Specific assumptions about nurse-client interactions are:

- Perceptions of nurse and of client influence the interaction process.
- Goals, needs, and values of nurse and client influence the interaction process.
- Individuals have a right to knowledge about themselves.
- Individuals have a right to participate in decisions that influence their life, their health, and community services.
- Health professionals have a responsibility to share information that helps individuals make informed decisions about their health care.
- Individuals have a right to accept or to reject health care.
- Goals of health professionals and goals of recipients of health care may be incongruent (King, pp. 143-144).

Concepts

The major concepts in the theory of goal attainment are interaction, perception, communication, transaction, self, role, stress, growth and development, time, and space. These 10 concepts have been theoretically defined to show the interrelationships among them. One of the concepts, transaction, has been operationally defined (King, 1981, pp. 150-151). The definitions are presented here.

DEFINITIONS OF THE CONCEPTS

1. *Interaction.* "A process of perception and communication between person and environment and between person and person, represented by verbal and non-verbal behaviors that are goal-directed." (King, 1981, p. 145)

2. *Perception.* "Each person's representation of reality. It is an awareness of persons, objects, and events." (King, 1981, p. 146)

3. *Communication.* "A process whereby information is given from one person to another either directly in face-to-face meetings or indirectly through telephone, television, or the written word. Communication is the information component of an interaction." (King, 1981, p. 146)

4. *Transaction.* Refer to the operational definition (p. 150-151). The conceptual definition is that transaction "is an observable behavior of human beings interacting with their environment. Transactions are viewed as the valuation component of human interaction." (King, 1981, p. 147)

5. *Role.* "A set of behaviors expected of persons occupying a position in a social system; rules that define rights and obligations in a position; a relationship with one or more individuals interacting in a specific situation for a purpose." (King, 1981, p. 147)

6. *Stress.* "A dynamic state whereby a human being interacts with the environment to maintain balance for growth, development and performance." (King, 1981, p. 147)

7. *Growth and development.* "Two distinct concepts used
together in most nursing and related literature. Together they
are defined as continuous changes in individuals at the cellu-
lar, molecular, and behavioral levels of activities." (King, 1981,
p. 148)

8. *Time.* "A sequence of events moving onward to the future. Time is a continuous flow of events in successive order
that implies change, a past, and a future. Time is a duration
between one event and another as uniquely experienced by
each human being; it is the relationship of one event to another." (King, 1981, p. 148)

9. *Self.* "A personal system defined as a unified, complex
whole; self who perceives, thinks, desires, imagines, decides,
identifies goals and selects means to achieve them." (King,
1981, p. 27)

10. *Space.* "Existing in all directions and the same every-
where. Space is a physical area called territory and is defined
by the behavior of individuals occupying space, such as ges-
tures, postures, and visible boundaries erected to mark off personal space." (King, 1981, p. 148)

Following Kerlinger's definition (1973), which delineates defined concepts as one of the elements in a theory, the next element
is a set of propositions that show some relationship among the
constructs (concepts) of the theory.

Propositions

The following directional propositions are selected from the
theory; others could be generated.

1. If perceptual accuracy is present in nurse-client interactions, transactions will occur.

2. If nurse and client make transactions, goals will be attained.

3. If goals are attained, effective nursing care will occur.

4. If transactions are made in nurse-client interactions, growth and development will be enhanced.

5. If role expectations and role performance as perceived by nurse and client are congruent, transactions will occur.

Identifying propositions from the theory is a continuous process. This usually occurs when one attempts to test the ideas of a theory in research. From propositions, one moves to research questions or to formulation of hypotheses that can be tested in research. The hypotheses stated here are different from those in the 1981 edition of King.

Hypotheses Generated From King's Theory

The hypotheses stated here are being tested in several ongoing research studies. These hypotheses evolve directly from the interrelationship of concepts in the theory of goal attainment.

1. Mutual goal setting will increase functional abilities in performing activities of daily living.

2. Mutual goal setting will increase elderly patients' morale.

3. Mutual goal setting by nurse and client leads to goal attainment.

4. Goal attainment will be greater in patients who participate in mutual goal setting than in patients who do not participate.

5. Role conflict between nurse and patient may increase stress in nursing situations.

These hypotheses suggest a few examples and nurses who read this theory may generate many more hypotheses to test in research.

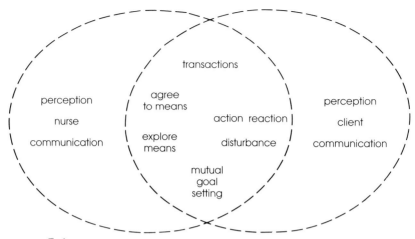

FIGURE 7-1
Theory of Goal Attainment. (From King, I. M.: A Theory For Nursing: Systems, Concepts, Process. New York, John Wiley & Sons, 1981, p. 157.)

HUMAN INTERACTION/TRANSACTION PROCESS

A model of nurse-patient interactions that lead to transactions was the result of a descriptive study of nurse-patient interactions using trained observers. An operational definition of transactions was formulated prior to conducting this descriptive study (King, 1981, pp. 150-151). The classification system for studying transactions that lead to goal attainment was derived from the interaction data. This study identified a nurse-patient interaction process that leads to transactions that leads to goal attainment. The findings were confirmed from analysis of interaction data in two other studies in which time series data were available. Analysis of time series nurse-patient interaction data confirmed the definition of a human interaction process that leads to mutual goal setting, transactions, and goal attainment in nursing situations.

A schematic diagram of the theory of goal attainment is shown in Figure 7-1.

Some of the concepts of the theory are implicit in this diagram such as role (nurse and client) and interaction. Work is in progress to develop a model to represent the theory.

Nursing is a construct just as health, government, stress, time, and space, and as a construct it is in need of data. Data come from the concrete world, so an operational definition of the construct is essential to collect data. The definition of nursing that can be used to generate data about the construct is: Nursing is a process of human interactions between nurse and client whereby each perceives the other and the situation, and through communications, they set goals, explore the means to achieve them, agree to the means, and their actions indicate movement toward goal achievement.

The interrelationship of theory and research must be the focus of our attention in the future. If nursing expects to be recognized as scientific by colleagues in other disciplines, nurse scholars should foster the idea that a theory has generated ideas that are tested in research and that the published findings show how nursing research is building knowledge for application in practice.

Remember that theory generates knowledge through research. It is important to conduct the research that is essential in building knowledge for nursing rather than to focus on application until knowledge from research is available for application in practice.

REFERENCES

Adams, E. (1985). Toward more clarity in terminology: Frameworks, theories and models. *Journal of Nursing Education*, *24*(4):151-155.

Kerlinger, F. N. (1973). *Foundations of behavioral research*. New York: Holt, Rinehart & Winston.

King, I. M. (1981). *A theory for nursing: Systems, concepts, process*. New York: John Wiley & Sons, pp. 141-161.

Reynolds, P. (1971). *A primer in theory construction*. Indianapolis, IN: The Bobbs-Merrill Co.

8

A Critique of King's Theory

SHARON J. MAGAN

The scientific tradition is lived among this community of scholars who value the activities and goals of science. Kaplan wrote that, "Science itself is a social enterprise, in which data are shared, ideas exchanged, and experiments replicated. It is precisely the cumulation of empirical evidence which shapes a wealth of diverse opinions into scientific knowledge common to many minds" (1964, p.36). These scientific activities include the scholarly exchange of ideas as well as a critical examination of ideas. The critique is a powerful tool for disciplined reflection and evaluation of theoretical formulations in light of criteria.

Structure

HISTORICAL EVOLUTION

King's theory of goal attainment (1981) describes a perspective of what is happening in nursing situations. It focuses on the process that occurs between a nurse and a client, which is initiated to help a client cope with a health problem that compromises the client's ability to maintain social roles, functions, and activities of daily living.

The roots of the theory of goal attainment appear in King's 1971 work, *Toward a Theory for Nursing*. Building on the work of Peplau (1952) and Orlando (1961), King (1971) has studied nursing process as a goal-directed interaction between nurses and clients. She wrote of Man in relation to the social structure of society and using four major concepts as a frame of reference for nursing practice. These concepts were social systems, perceptions, interpersonal relations, and health. King (1971) explained the relationship among the concepts; she indicated that Man functions in social systems through interpersonal relationships in terms of perceptions which influence life and health. The framework for the early development of the theory was social systems or networks of interacting systems, which is not to be confused with the general system theory of von Bertalanffy (1968). King developed the concepts of transaction, perception, and communication to explain what happens in the nursing process.

The theory of goal attainment uses some of the same concepts identified in King's 1971 work. This most recent work is based overall on the concepts of human beings, environment, health, and society, as opposed to social systems, perception, interpersonal relations and health in the earlier work.

PHILOSOPHICAL ASSUMPTIONS

The theory of goal attainment is structured with explicit philosophical assumptions related to Man and the nurse-client interaction. King identified nine separate assumptions related to Man, which are written in single statements, with one word descriptors: individuals are social, sentient, rational, reacting, perceiving, controlling, purposeful, action oriented, and time oriented (King, 1981, p.143). These assumptions are written at more of a concrete level than a philosophical level and provide a list of descriptions without specifying any kind of relationship between them.

There are also specific assumptions about nurse-client interactions in this theory:

1. Individuals have a right to knowledge about themselves.

2. Individuals have the right to participate in decisions that influence their life, their health, and community services.

3. Individuals have a right to accept or to reject health care (p. 143).

These assumptions are stated in terms of the individual rights to knowledgeable participation in health care decision-making and might be combined in one general assumption written in more abstract terms to cover more situations.

The remaining assumptions are concerned with the interaction process between nurse and client (King, 1981, p. 143). One of these assumptions states that the "Perceptions of nurse and of client influence the interaction process." Perception and interaction are major concepts in the theoretical framework that are related to each other in King's concept development. This statement might be addressed as a proposition rather than an assumption. The last assumption states that, "Goals, needs, and values of nurse and client influence the interaction process." While it is written in operational terms rather than philosophical terms, it does represent an assumption on which the transaction concept is further developed in the framework.

PRINCIPLES, CONCEPTS, AND PROPOSITIONS

The structure of the theory of goal attainment includes no principles, only major concepts derived from an explicitly stated conceptual framework. While this theory does not offer principles, it does include a statement that refers to postulated ideas. A brief statement outlining a definition of nursing describes the overall theory of goal attainment: "Nursing is a process of human interactions between nurse and client whereby each perceives the other and the situation; and through communication, they set goals, explore means, and agree on means to achieve goals" (King, 1981, p. 144). There are also eight stated propositions and seven hypotheses that specify more about the theory.

DEFINITION OF MAN

In the theory of goal attainment, King refers to Man as a human being or an individual, which is different from her 1971 work in which she discussed Man as a human organism. The explicitly stated assumptions provided descriptions of Man as social, sentient, rational, reacting, perceiving, controlling, purposeful, action oriented and time oriented (King, 1981, p. 143). King (1981, p. 10) also stated a basic premise of her work is that "human beings are open systems interacting with environment." However, King's concept of Man as an open system is derived from a social systems perspective that should not be confused with the general system perspective of von Bertalanffy (1968), who used the concepts of wholeness, negentropy, equifinality, and pattern and organization to describe open systems. Although King described Man as an open system, her assumptions that describe Man as reacting and controlling suggest a way of responding to stimuli without the mutuality that marks an open system perspective.

King (1981, p. 141) also characterized Man as a total person when she wrote that "a major thesis of the framework is that each human being perceives the world as a total person in making transactions with individuals and things in the environment." In another place in her work, King stated that "individuals react as total human beings to their experiences, which are viewed as a flow of events in time" (1981, p. 20). While these statements do not appear as stated assumptions, they do reflect a philosophical perspective about Man as a totality.

DEFINITION OF HEALTH

King's concept of health tells more about her view of human beings. "Health is defined as dynamic life experiences of a human being, which implies continuous adjustment to stressors in the internal and external environment through optimum use of one's resources to achieve maximum potential for daily living. Illness is defined as a deviation from normal, that is, an imbalance in a person's biological structure or in his psychological make-up, or a conflict in a person's social relationships" (King, 1981, p. 5). The emphasis is on understanding Man's health through reference to difficulties in specific parts, rather than a wholeness perspective of Man which pervades other nursing theories. King's view of Man and health is consistent with the totality paradigm.

King (1981) also referred to health as a state that marks an individual's ability to function in social roles. The earlier reference to health as dynamic life experiences implies a process orientation that conflicts with the idea of health as a state. Health cannot logically be both a state and a process. The continuous adjustment to stressors in the internal and external environment implies an adaptation process that is also reflective of the totality paradigm.

King's idea of health from the social interaction perspective, which posits health as an ability to function in social roles, is not developed in relation to the quality of functioning in social roles. Instead, indicators of health are discussed in relation to mortality, morbidity, standards of living, accidents, and environmental factors—areas more consistent with an idea of health as the absence of disease. King has suggested that nurses consider the use of epidemiological methods to "identify factors in communities that relate to health promotion" (1981, p. 6).

The difficulty with a consistent understanding of health in King's framework is further complicated by her assertion that health and disease do not constitute polarities, while she also maintained that illness is an interference or disturbance in health. If health is indeed "dynamic life experiences of a human being including continuous adjustment to stressors in the internal and external environment" (King, 1981, p. 5), then illness or disease is not an interference or disturbance but rather that which is involved in the adjustment process, not something separate and outside of it.

King stated that, "The goal of nursing is to help individuals and groups attain, maintain, and restore health" (1981, p.13). If health represents continual dynamic life experiences, then it can never be absent or lost, but is merely different, depending on how an individual experiences self in the environment.

This theory is specifically limited to the processes involved in the nurse-client interaction toward health. It is concerned with how nursing care is given in relation to how needs and goals are identified. King set the stage for this activity when she proposed boundaries for her theory. Boundaries indicate the context in which the theory is applicable (Kaplan, 1964, pp. 95-96). Most of the interior boundary criteria are concerned with identifying who is considered to be a nurse and who is a client; for example, a nurse is a licensed professional with special skills. It does not seem necessary to make this kind of distinction. The fifth criterion appears to be the most significant in terms of specifying the context for the theory. It states that "Nurse and client are in mutual presence, purposefully interacting to achieve goals" (King, 1981, p. 150). This statement indicates that application of this particular theory cannot be delegated to others because it is contingent on "mutual presence" (p. 150) of nurse and client.

Exterior boundary criteria in the theory for King include interactions in a two-person group. This criterion specifies the number of individuals involved in a nurse-client interaction in which the theory applies. In that King limited the boundaries of the theory to interaction in a two-person group, it appears that this theory would not be appropriate for a family-centered nursing practice or community group practice. The third exterior boundary criterion states that interactions take place in natural environments. Since King argued that "nurse-client interactions can occur in any nursing situation at any time or in any place" (p. 150), the meaning of "natural" environments is not clear.

In the summary of the theory of goal attainment, King (1981) proposed another assumption related to health in general that is not listed with the philosophical assumptions. She stated that "There is a basic assumption in the theory presented, that is, that generally patients and nurses communicate information, mutually set goals, and take action to attain goals" (1981, p. 157). This statement is referred to as a basic assumption but is actually another way of stating the meaning of the theory itself as it was discussed in the introduction to the theory in the following statements: "This theory describes the nature of nurse-client interactions that lead to achievement of goals. It presents a standard for nurse-patient interactions, namely, that nurses purposefully interact with clients mutually to establish goals and to explore and agree on means to achieve goals. Mutual goal setting is based on nurses' assessment of clients' concerns, problems, and disturbances in health, their perception to move toward goal attainment (pp. 142-143). It is confusing to see the same ideas referred to as an assumption and as a description of the theory itself.

RELATIONSHIP BETWEEN MAN AND HEALTH

Although King posits health as the goal of nursing, the link between Man and health is not well forged in the description of the conceptual framework and theoretical formulation. Health is not specifically related to the development of any of the major concepts in the framework, nor is it dealt with per se in the propositions or hypotheses. For example, although the concepts of growth and development are defined as "processes that take place in the life of individuals that help them move from potential capacity for achievement to self-actualization" (1981, p. 148), they are not explicitly linked to health.

Process

CORRESPONDENCE

Established Knowledge of Man and Health

King's basic views of Man and health are consistent with those of Neuman (1982). Like Neuman, King (1981) described Man as a total person who is goal oriented and purposeful and reacts to stressors. Both Neuman and King discussed Man as an open system, but neither developed the critical concepts of negentropy and wholeness as more than the sum of parts in relation to Man as an open system. Both theorists accounted for individual differences in people and agree that perception of stressors and events vary from one individual to another. Both theorists also acknowledged illness as a description. Neuman (1982, p. 10) stated that "illness is a state of insufficiency, disrupting needs are yet to be satisfied." King (1981, p. 5) proposed that "illness indicates some interferences in the (life) cycle." King's concept of health centers on the continuous adjustment to internal and external stressors for maximum functioning within the context of human growth and development. This conception of health coincides with homeostatic, and adaptational perspectives of health and disease. The theory of goal attainment is related to established knowledge concerning instrumental interactions in social systems.

Interrelation of Concepts at Same Level of Discourse

The theory of goal attainment is based on a conceptual framework containing three major concepts: personal systems, interpersonal systems, and social systems. The concept of personal systems has six subconcepts, including perception, self, growth and development, body image, space, and time. The concept of interpersonal systems has five subconcepts, including human interaction, communication, transactions, role, and stress. The concept of social systems has five subconcepts, including organization, authority, power, status, and decision-making.

Despite the presence of three main concepts in this framework, the theory of goal attainment is based on only one of these concepts, that of interpersonal systems, and now that concept subsumes 10 subconcepts instead of the original 5. The other five subconcepts were borrowed from the other two major concepts, personal and social systems, which, despite their previous significance in the conceptual framework, are summarized or incorporated into interpersonal systems. The organization of concepts affects the logical structure and flow of ideas so that the meaning of the concepts signifying three interacting systems becomes somewhat confused when one system, the interpersonal, subsumes some concepts of the other two systems, personal and social systems.

An examination of the flow of ideas from the conceptual framework to the theoretical framework reveals an inconsistency in the number of concepts that are treated and the levels of discourse. For example, 10 major concepts are listed in the theory of goal attainment, but only 9 are defined. The concept of self was not defined at this point in the theory. This inconsistency and the difficulty with logical structures weakens the pattern of relatedness that the theory has with extant knowledge and the internal pattern of relatedness through which the meaning of the theory is enhanced.

The clarity of meaning in the theory is jeopardized by definitions of concepts that are indistinct, so that it is difficult to differentiate one concept from another. For example, in the larger conceptual framework, King (1981) suggested common characteristics of perception that help to define perception (p. 22), and included a statement that "Perception is transaction" (p. 23)—an addition that confuses both concepts. In addition, she discussed perception as both a thing that is perceived (that is, "each human being's representation of reality," p. 20), and as a "process of organizing, interpreting and transforming information from sense data and memory" (p. 24). Meaning is clarified when concepts are consistently discussed from the same perspective.

The logical relationships between the concepts are strengthened when all of the concepts selected share some feature in common. For example, transaction, interaction, communication, and perception could all be developed from a process perspective. The concept of role as a function does not fit semantically with the process concepts.

King (1981) referred to the concept of stress as both a process and a factor that affects a process, or a "stressor." King's definition of stress as "a dynamic state whereby a human being interacts with the environment to maintain balance for growth, development, and performance" (p. 147) is not consistent with general approaches to the concept of stress as a coping process that requires adjustment in perspectives, activities, and lifestyles.

The clarity and meaning of the theory of goal attainment might be enhanced by concentrating on the four concepts—communication, perception, interaction, and transaction—that share a process orientation without involving additional concepts. The additional concepts of growth and development, time, and space are at a higher level of discourse than the other five concepts. These concepts refer to broader processes with more encompassing dimensions. King (1981) described the concept of space in the framework as a discrete territory that is significant in relation to how individuals perceive space and use space to communicate their needs (p. 148). In this context, space might be more appropriately addressed in relation to the concepts of perception and communication. While King (1981) did discuss the concept of time in relation to rhythmicity in circadian patterns, duration, and succession, it was referred to in a postulated statement as a context in which stressors affect nurse-client interaction. King (1981) briefly discussed time in relation to perception, and like space, it might be addressed in relation to perception rather than as a separate concept. Although time and space were referred to together in postulated statement, King (1981) discussed them separately, which is consistent with the totality paradigm that expresses that time and space are indeed separate entities.

The concepts of health, human beings, environment, and society were presented as the overall abstract concepts represented in this framework, yet health and society do not directly relate to the 10 major concepts nor to the postulated statement, propositions, or hypotheses that describe the theory. An oblique reference to health can be found in a general description of the theory of goal attainment when King (1981) wrote of "mutual goal setting based on the nurses' assessment of client's concerns, problems and disturbances in health" (p. 142). It is surprising that, given the social systems framework for analysis of nurse-client interaction, no concepts were selected that directly relate to society or social systems. While the theory is limited to understanding dyadic interaction as specified in the boundary criteria, utilization of the concept of power might enhance an understanding of goal attainment in the nurse-client interaction.

Relationship to Paradigmatic Perspectives and Philosophical Assumptions

King's philosophical assumptions about Man and major concepts refer to a mechanistic, adaptational perspective that is consistent with the totality paradigm as opposed to the simultaneity paradigm (Parse and others, 1985). Man is described as a controlling, reacting, social being who is also rational, purposeful, time-oriented and action oriented. There is no reference to creative processes that transcend the rational. Although time and space were referred to together in King's postulational statement, King discussed them separately, which is consistent with the totality paradigm in which time and space are indeed separate entities.

King's assumptions about nurse-client interactions included the clients' right to participate in decisions that influence their life and health and to accept or reject health care. However, the nurse retains authority for providing information in health care decision making according to King's interior boundary criteria (1981, p. 150), coinciding with values of the totality paradigm.

King's focus on health as adjustment to stressors in growth and development processes leading to a state in which individuals demonstrate abilities to function in social roles indicates that health is related to norms congruent with the totality paradigm in which health is viewed as a deviation from the norm.

Description and Meaning of Principles, Concepts, and Propositions

King (1981) did not strictly designate principles flowing from her assumptions, but she postulated a statement that emphasizes the importance of the concepts of interaction, communication, transaction, role, and stress. She wrote, "It is postulated that nurse and client interactions are characterized by verbal and nonverbal communication, in which information is exchanged and interpreted; by transactions, in which values, needs, and wants of each member of the dyad are shared; by perception of nurse and client and the situation; by self in role of client and self in role of nurse; and by stressors influencing each person and the situation in time and space" (p. 142). Five separate postulational statements might be organized to enhance the clarity of these ideas.

King conceived eight propositions that further describe the theory of goal attainment (King, 1981, p. 149). The first proposition states that "if perceptual accuracy is present in the nurse-client interactions, transactions will occur" (King, 1981, p. 149). This proposition contains abstract terms that appropriately relate to the theoretical framework of the theory. Perceptual accuracy is more specific than perception but remains at a high enough level of abstraction to permit more concrete specification in the process of operationalizing for testing.

The second proposition states that "if nurse and client make transactions, goals will be attained" (King, 1981, p. 149). There is a problem with this proposition since transaction was defined in the conceptual framework as goal attainment (King, 1981, p. 61). Essentially then, this statement does not relate two different ideas but is concerned with only one. The if-then construction is misleading and the meaning is not clear. In addition, the idea of goal attainment is actually the whole theory. A more specific concept specifying priorities in goal attainment or satisfaction might be developed to reflect the larger construct of goal attainment.

The third proposition says that "if goals are attained, satisfactions will occur" (King, 1981, p. 149). It is natural to expect that attaining goals that reflect individuals' values provides a sense of satisfaction. However, even though transaction is defined as goal attainment, it is also concerned with the processes of bargaining, negotiating, and sharing that do not always result in the attainment of goals.

The fourth proposition states that "if goals are attained, effective nursing care will occur" (King, 1981, p. 149). This proposition is stated in very concrete terms and also appears as a circular statement. If the nurse and patient have mutually identified goals in the process of transaction, then it follows that these goals would represent effective nursing care.

The fifth proposition states that "if transactions are made in nurse-client interactions, growth and development will be enhanced" (King, 1981, p. 149). This is quite a departure from the concrete terms that were used in the fourth proposition. However, this proposition is also problematic, since it involves a statement that attempts to bridge a large gap between concepts at very different levels of discourse. To move from what happens in a transaction as values are shared in a nurse-patient interaction to the large process of growth and development marks a large conceptual leap through time and levels of abstraction.

The sixth proposition states that "if role expectations and role performance as perceived by nurse and client are congruent, transactions will occur" (King, 1981, p. 149). Role expectation and role performance are rooted in the concept of role that is part of the theoretical framework. These concepts of role performance and role conflict are sufficiently abstract to permit movement down the levels of abstraction for testing.

The seventh proposition states that "if role conflict is experienced by nurse or client or both, stress in nurse-client interactions will occur" (King, 1981, p. 149). Role conflict can be directly related to the concept of role in the framework while stress is a concept in the framework.

The eighth proposition states that "if nurses with special knowledge and skills communicate appropriate information to clients, mutual goal setting and goal attainment will occur" (King, 1981, p. 149). This proposition emphasizes the importance of a certain kind of communication on transactions. It is derived from communication and transaction which are explicitly stated concepts in the framework. However, it is at a lower level of discourse and sounds more like a hypothesis.

While there is some difficulty with some of the concreteness of terms in the propositions, an overall examination of the propositions indicates that they are logically related to the conceptual framework. All of the propositions are focused on the nurse-client interaction, which is the heart of the nursing process in this theory. The theory was put forth as an explanation for what happens in nursing situations in terms of how care is given. King remained true to her purpose in developing propositions that focus on this process.

King also offered seven hypotheses that were derived from the theory. These hypotheses should reflect a slightly lower level of abstraction than the propositions but are actually very similar except that they do not use a universal propositional if-then construction. The first hypothesis states that "perceptual accuracy in nurse-patient interactions increases mutual goal setting" (King, 1981, p.156). This hypothesis coincides with the first proposition but specifies transaction as mutual goal setting. Perceptual accuracy might be further specified here at a lower level of abstraction like, validation of perception increases mutual goal setting.

The second hypothesis, "communication increases goal setting between nurses and patients and leads to satisfactions" (King, 1981, p. 156). This hypothesis does not coincide with or conflict with any of King's propositions (1981, p. 149). The eighth proposition does state that "if nurses with special knowledge and skills communicate appropriate information to clients, mutual goal setting and goal attainment will occur." Communication is one of the major concepts of the theory of goal attainment.

The third hypothesis states that "satisfactions in nurses and patients increase goal attainment" (King, 1981, p. 156). This hypothesis is the mirror image of proposition 3 (King, 1981, p. 149), which was discussed earlier as a circular statement. By changing the direction of the concepts in this hypothesis, King was suggesting something else. She asserted that the more satisfactions nurses and clients experience, the more goals they will obtain. Satisfaction is discussed in relation to pleasurable outcomes from meeting valued goals and is only loosely related to the concept of transaction.

The fourth hypothesis states that "goal attainment decreases stress and anxiety in nursing situations" (King, 1981, p. 156). This proposition introduces a concept that has not been dealt with explicitly until now: anxiety. The semantic integrity of the framework would be enhanced by staying with the idea of stress and not introducing a topic that has not been specifically addressed and may connote several meanings.

The fifth hypothesis states that "goal attainment increases patient learning and coping ability in nursing situations" (King, 1981, p. 156). Patient learning and coping abilities do not have a specific root. These concepts might be linked to health and learning as a way of coping in social roles. Explicating a relationship such as this might even strengthen the meaning of the theoretical structure.

The sixth hypothesis states that "role conflict experienced by patients, nurses or both, decreases transactions in nurse-patient interactions" (King, 1981, p.156). Role conflict is suitable for testing at the level of a hypothesis while transaction should be further specified in a more concrete manner.

The seventh hypothesis states that "congruence in role expectations and role performance increases transactions in nurse-patient interactions" (King, 1981, p. 156). The concept of role is linked to transaction in this hypothesis too with role congruence in terms of both expectations and performances leading to further specification appropriate for hypothetical formulation while transaction remains at a propositional level.

There are difficulties in relation to internal consistency and logical structuring of ideas in the theory of goal attainment. However, King designed this theory to explain what happens in nursing situations in relation to how care is given. King remained true to her purpose in developing a postulated statement, propositions, and hypotheses that focus on this process.

COHERENCE

Relation of Theory to Other Theories

The theory of goal attainment extends the work of Orlando (1961), Henderson (1955), and Peplau (1952), who focused on the nurse-patient relations and as such fits a certain tradition in nursing's development that has to do with what happens between the nurse and the patient in the process of giving care aimed at maintaining or restoring health. The theory of goal attainment focuses on how the nurse gives care while the what of care or nursing content is relegated to a synthesis of principles, concepts, laws, and theories from the natural and social sciences (King, 1971, p. 3). This focus on how to give care belongs to the nursing process tradition within the discipline of nursing which is concerned with the nurse's way of identifying the client's needs and meeting those needs through systematic planning and evaluation with whatever resources are at the nurse's disposal. King has written that "nursing is a process of human interactions between nurse and client in which each perceives and communicates with the other to set goals, explore means, and agree on means to achieve goals" (1981, p. 144). This view of nursing coincides with that of Peplau (1952, p. 5), who viewed nursing as a therapeutic, goal-directed interpersonal process. King's view of nursing is also related to that of Orlando (1961), whose principles of nursing practice reflect specific ways of ascertaining patient's needs through exploration and validation of what and how the nurse and patient communicate with each other.

Logical Flow from Assumptions to Propositions

There are difficulties in relation to internal consistency and logical structuring of ideas in the theory of goal attainment. The nine major concepts of the theory are rooted in both personal systems and interpersonal systems in the conceptual framework. However, all are subsumed under interpersonal systems in the description of the theory of goal attainment. The logical flow of ideas in the framework is hindered by the discussion of concepts at different levels of discourse. For example, growth and development is discussed on the same level as communication and role. There is a logical relationship between major concepts and propositions, but the concreteness of some terms in the propositions (role conflict), along with higher level abstractions (transactions), detracts somewhat from the flow of ideas. The refinement of the propositions may also strengthen the logical flow of ideas by eliminating goal attainment as a concept from these statements. The overall theory should not be referred to as a concept as well.

Symmetry and Aesthetics

The aesthetic value of a theory is enhanced by its simplicity, power, and balance that rest on logical structuring and clarity. At present the theory of goal attainment lacks a symmetrical quality in the range of concepts treated, their various levels of discourse, and the lack of propositions that relate to all of the major concepts. Symmetry might be enhanced by selecting process-oriented concepts such as communication, interaction, and transaction, and developing specific propositions that relate these concepts to each other.

Another set of concepts with interrelating principles might also be developed such as role, stress, and perception. These sets of concepts and their principles might be related to each other through another set of principles. This type of logical structuring enhances the aesthetic dimension of the theory by creating a symmetry in ideas and coherence that adds power to the network of concepts explained in the theory.

PRAGMATICS

Use of Theory in Practice and Research

It is disappointing that implications for practice that center on the use of the concepts in process are overshadowed by King's contention that a goal-oriented nursing record "will help nurses increase their skills in making nursing diagnoses, in verifying accuracy in perceptions, in purposeful nurse-client interactions, and in helping individuals participate in making decisions that influence their life and their health" (1981, p. 172). King (1981) has asserted that the goal list of a nursing record will help the nurse "monitor disturbances or interferences in patients" (p. 171). The theory of goal attainment that describes a process of interaction is not explicitly related to this nursing record. In fact, King used a conceptual approach to discuss the importance of the nursing record that was not related to any of the ideas she had previously discussed. The conceptual basis of the Goal-Oriented Nursing Record (GONR) was the problem-oriented medical record espoused by Weed (1969). Implications or guidelines for nursing intervention can be derived from King's propositions and hypotheses. Nurses should be cognizant of many variables that are present in any individual nurse-client interaction. This would enhance the accuracy of the nurses' perception of the clients' perception of health care situation and would promote the occurrence of transactions. It behooves the nurse to explore ways of enhancing perceptual accuracy, and ways of structuring situations with clients in order to attend to ways of examining and verifying perceptual accuracy. King's propositions also suggest the importance of nurses explicitly sharing the specific purpose in being with a particular client in a particular nursing situation. In addition to clarifying the purpose of the nurse-client interaction, nurses might specifically examine expectations related to their roles with clients. These practice implications are directly related to ideas discussed in the propositions and hypotheses yet not specified by King. There are no specific published reports of King's theory as used in practice.

The research testing the hypothesis that "communication increases mutual goal setting between nurses and patients and leads to satisfactions" (King, 1981, p. 156), will require further development of this hypothesis. Communication is too large a concept to be treated without qualification in a hypothesis. Many facets of communications might be examined. The kinds of communication might be investigated according to its relevance for both nurse and client. What kinds of information are clients interested in? How does the nurse choose a style of communicating that fits the kind of information that is dealt with and the style of the client? Are the nurses' satisfactions different from or conflictual with the clients'? How does this relate to goal attainment especially in regard to the issues of clients' compliance with treatment? These questions point toward the many directions that could be pursued in working with the fifth hypothesis.

Further development of the theory of goal attainment would be enhanced by tightening the internal structure of the theory and further specifying the interrelationship of the concepts in relation to explicit principles. This would provide more direction for the generation of propositions and testable hypotheses. There are no specific published reports of research related to King's theory.

Contribution to Nursing Science

King's theory of goal attainment has made a significant contribution to nursing science by offering a conceptual approach to nursing process that moves beyond a strict observational and problem-solving approach. The utility of theory is enhanced by its focus on the helping relationships so that it is possible that this theory could be applied with other nursing theories from the same paradigmatic totality perspective. For example, the theory of goal attainment might be used in conjunction with Roy's Adaptation Model as a way of enhancing the collection of data about the adaptive modes of physiological needs, self-concept, role function, and interdependence.

King's theory of goal attainment provides the discipline of nursing with a theoretical base for applying the traditional nursing process. The value of King's work for nursing theory-based practice will continue to enhance the scientific progress of the discipline of nursing.

REFERENCES

Henderson, V. (1955). The nature of nursing. Reprinted in M. E. Meyers, ed, *Nursing fundamentals.* Dubuque, IA: William C. Brown Co.

Kaplan, A. (1964). *The conduct of inquiry.* Scranton: Chandler Publishing Co.

King, I. M. (1971). *Toward a theory for nursing.* New York: John Wiley & Sons.

King, I. M. (1978). The why of theory development. *In Theory development: What, why, how?* New York: National League for Nursing, pp. 11-16.

King, I. M. (1981). *A theory for nursing: Systems, concepts, process.* New York: John Wiley & Sons.

Neuman, B. (1982). *The Neuman systems model.* Norwalk, CT: Appleton-Century-Crofts.

Orlando, I. J. (1961). *The dynamic nurse-patient relationship.* New York: G. P. Putnam's Sons.

Parse, R. R., Coyne, A. B., and Smith, M. J. (1985). *Nursing research: Qualitative methods.* Bowie, MD: Brady Communications.

Peplau, H. (1952). *Interpersonal relations in nursing.* New York: G. P. Putnam's Sons.

von Bertalanffy, L. (1968). *General system theory.* New York: George Braziller.

Weed, L. L. (1969). *Medical records, medical education, and patient care.* Cleveland, OH: Case Western Reserve University Press.

SECTION OVERVIEW
The Simultaneity Paradigm

ROSEMARIE RIZZO PARSE

The Man-environment simultaneity paradigm is an
alternative to the traditional predominant worldview in
nursing. This paradigm evolved as a new view in the
early 1970's (Rogers, 1970). It, like the totality
paradigm, is rooted in one view of Nightingale's works. It
is natural in the evolution of a discipline to spawn
different paradigms as scientists within a field venture
outside the operating belief system to describe and
explain phenomena. The beliefs set forth in the
simultaneity paradigm moved nursing away from a
particulate view of Man toward a view that, for nursing,
entirely reframed Man as more than and different from
the sum of the parts. The simultaneity paradigm is
gaining in recognition among scientists in nursing, and is
beginning to have an impact on research and practice
competitive with the totality paradigm.

The simultaneity paradigm differs from the totality

paradigm in three significant ways: in the assumptions about Man and health, in the goals of nursing, and in the implications for research and practice.

Assumptions About Man and Health

In the simultaneity paradigm, Man is viewed as more than and different from the sum of the parts (Parse and others, 1985). Man is an open being free to choose in mutual rhythmical interchange with the environment. Man gives meaning to situations and is responsible for choices in moving beyond what is (Parse, 1981). Man and the environment are recognized by their respective patterns. Man lives in a relative Now experiencing the what was, is, and will be, all at once. Health is viewed as a process of becoming and as a set of value priorities. Health is Man's unfolding. It is experienced by the individual and can only be described by that individual. There is no optimum health; health is simply how one is experiencing personal living.

The theoretical roots broadly related to the simultaneity view are grounded in the works of de Chardin (1965), von Bertalanffy (1968), Polanyi (1958), Sartre (1963), Heidegger (1962), Merleau-Ponty (1963), and Einstein (1946). The language of the theories in this paradigm is specified at a level that adds different dimensions and possibilities to the science of nursing. The conceptualizations are systematized structures unique to nursing science.

Goals of Nursing

The goals of nursing in the simultaneity paradigm focus on quality of life from the person's perspective. Nursing is practiced with all individuals and families. Designation of illness by societal norms is not a significant factor. Parse's theory in this paradigm guides practice that focuses on illuminating meaning and moving beyond the moment with the person and family relative to changing health patterns (Parse, 1981). The authority figure and prime decision maker in regard to nursing is the person, not the nurse. There are no systematized nursing care plans based on health problems. The person in the nurse-person interrelationship determines the activities for changing health patterns; the nurse in true presence with the person guides the way (Parse, 1981). The outcomes of nursing practice in this paradigm are described by the person in light of that individual's own plans for changing health patterns as they relate to quality of life.

Implications for Research and Practice

Nursing research that is related to the theories from the simultaneity paradigm is generally qualitative in nature. Since the early 1970's some quantitative research methods have been used to study phenomena in this paradigm (Rogers, 1970). This was done at a time when qualitative methods were viewed as nonscientific and thus unacceptable as a mode of scientific inquiry. The qualitative methods borrowed from the social and human sciences are consistent with the beliefs about Man in the simultaneity paradigm and have been used to enhance theories (Parse and others, 1985). These methods are appropriate while nursing science is developing. Unique methods of inquiry for nursing from the simultaneity paradigm perspective are being developed. An emerging methodology for Parse's theory has been created. It was derived directly from the theory itself and is unique to nursing science (Parse, 1986).

Nursing practice based on the theories in the simultaneity paradigm is beginning to be operationalized. The practice methodologies unique to the theories and the paradigm are being tested. As used in the totality paradigm, the nursing process of assessing, diagnosing, planning, implementing, and evaluating is not consistent with the beliefs of this paradigm and is thus inappropriate as a systematic mode of practice. The practice methodology for Parse's theory (1981) has been developed and focuses on illuminating meaning, synchronizing rhythms, and mobilizing transcendence with persons and families as a guide to changing health patterns in relationship to their personal quality of life.

Rogers (1970, 1980) and Parse (1981) creatively synthesized structures consistent with beliefs about Man and health in the simultaneity paradigm to guide research and practice. The chapters that follow are original works by these theorists describing the essences of their theories. Following each theory chapter is a critique using the criteria set forth in Chapter 1.

REFERENCES

de Chardin, T. (1965). *The phenomenon of man*. New York: Paulist Press.

Einstein, A. (1946). *The meaning of relativity*. Princeton: Princeton University Press.

Heidegger, M. (1962). *Being and time*. New York: Harper & Row.

Merleau-Ponty, M. (1963). *The structure of behavior*. Boston: Beacon Press.

Nightingale, F. (1969). *Notes on nursing: What it is and what it is not*. New York: Dover Publications. (Unabridged republication of the first American edition, as published in 1860 by D. Appleton & Company.)

Parse, R. R. (1981). *Man-living-health: A theory of nursing*. New York: John Wiley & Sons.

Parse, R. R., Coyne, A. B., and Smith, M. J. (1985). *Nursing research: Qualitative methods*. Bowie, MD: Brady Communications.

Parse, R. R. (1986). An emerging methodology for the Man-Living-Health theory. Unpublished manuscript. Pittsburgh, PA, Discovery International, Inc.

Polanyi, M. (1958). *Personal knowledge*. Chicago: University of Chicago Press.

Rogers, M. E. (1970) *An introduction to the theoretical basis of nursing*. Philadelphia: F. A. Davis Co.

Rogers, M. E. (1980) Nursing: A science of unitary man. *In* Riehl, J. P. and Roy, C., eds. *Conceptual models for nursing practice*. New York: Appleton-Century-Crofts.

Sartre, J. P. (1963). *Search for a method*. New York: Alfred A. Knopf.

von Bertalanffy, L. (1968). *General system theory*. New York: George Braziller.

Rogers's Science of Unitary Human Beings

MARTHA E. ROGERS

EDITORIAL PERSPECTIVE

Rogers (1970; 1980) describes Man and environment as energy fields in mutual interaction with each other. She believes this mutual interaction occurs simultaneously and thus negates cause-and-effect processes, a view consistent with the simultaneity paradigm. In fact, Rogers (1970) was the first to propose a nursing science base with Man and environment viewed in this way. Rogers (1970) views health as Man's becoming. The language of her framework reveals her belief that the open energy interchange between Man and environment creates distinct patterns by which each can be recognized. Rogers (1980) also posits four-dimensionality as a nonlinear domain without spatial or temporal attributes.

In the following pages, Rogers specifies the broad princi-

ples of the science of unitary Man, and makes explicit her beliefs about Man and environment.

━━━

   The uniqueness of nursing, like that of any other science, lies in
the phenomenon central to its purposes. Nursing's long-established
concern with human beings and their world is a natural forerunner
of an organized abstract system encompassing people and their environments. The irreducible nature of individuals as different from the
sum of parts and the integralness of human beings and environment
coordinate with a universe of open systems identifies the focus of a
new paradigm and initiates nursing's identity as a science.
   Nursing as a learned profession is both a science and an art
(Rogers, 1970, 1980). A science may be defined as an organized
body of abstract knowledge arrived at by scientific research and logical analysis. It has many principles and theories derived from conceptual systems. A science can have more than one paradigm or
conceptual system, but the phenomena of concern remain constant.
A worldview is a paradigm from which one can derive principles and
theories that can guide practice and enable better service to people.
The art of nursing is the imaginative and creative use of this knowledge in human service. Historically, the term nursing most often has
been used as a verb signifying "to do." When nursing is perceived as
a science, the term nursing becomes a noun signifying "a body of
abstract knowledge." The education of nurses transmits nursing's theoretical knowledge. The practice by nurses is the use of this knowledge in service to people. Research in nursing is the study of unitary
human beings and their environments.
   The introduction of systems theories several decades ago set
in motion new ways of perceiving people and their world. Science
and technology escalated. The exploration of space revised old
views. New knowledge merged with new ways of thinking. A second industrial revolution was initiated—far more dramatic in its
implications and potentials than the first. A pressing need to study
people in ways that would enhance their humanness coordinate
with accelerating technological advances forced a search for new
models. A major hindrance to evolving viable models, however,
was noted by Capra (1982) when he talked about trying to apply

concepts of an outdated worldview to a reality that can no longer be understood in terms of these concepts.

Beliefs About Human Beings and Environment

A science of unitary human beings basic to nursing requires a new worldview and a conceptual system specific to nursing's phenomena of concern. Peoples and their environments are perceived as irreducible energy fields integral with one another and continuously creative in their evolution. The proposed paradigm is humanistic, not mechanistic. Moreover, this is an optimistic model though not a utopian one. Further it is postulated that people have the capacity to participate knowingly and probabilistically in the process of change.

Unitary human beings are specified to be irreducible wholes. Moreover, a whole cannot be understood when it is reduced to its particulars. Unitary human beings are not to be confused with current popular usage of the term holistic, which generally signifies a summation of parts, whether few or many. A science of unitary human beings is unique to nursing as well as having relevance for other fields. The explication of a body of abstract knowledge concerning unitary persons requires an organized conceptual system from which to derive unifying principles and hypothetical generalizations basic to description, explanation, and prediction.

The development of a conceptual system is a process of the creative synthesis of facts and ideas out of which a new product emerges. Theories derive from the system and are tested in the real world. The findings of research are fed back into the system whereby the system undergoes continuous alteration, revision, and change. Certainly, the conceptual system and what comes out of it is not derived from any of the basic sciences of any other field. Nursing is not based on any of these; rather, it has its own unique irreducible mix. The parts cannot be removed or changed around or revised without altering the system. This conceptual system is the peculiar synthesis that has led to the product called the science of unitary human beings. Four building blocks for the paradigm are postulated, namely: energy field, a universe of open systems, pattern and four-dimensionality.

Building Blocks

Energy fields are postulated to constitute the fundamental unit of the living and the nonliving. Energy is defined in its general language sense as something that is dynamic. Field is a unifying concept and thus a dynamic unity. Energy signifies the dynamic nature of the field. Energy fields are infinite. Two energy fields are identified: the human field and the environmental field. Specifically, human beings and environment *are* energy fields. They do not have energy fields. The human and environmental fields are not biological, physical, social, or psychological fields; they are irreducible. Viewing unitary human beings as irreducible wholes is not a denial of knowledge about other things, meaning parts. But one cannot generalize from a field such as biology or psychology to unitary human beings. What may be very valid in describing biological phenomena does not describe unitary human beings, any more than describing a molecule tells you about laughter. Fields are abstraction.

A *universe of open systems* explains the infinite nature of energy fields; they are continuously open. The human and environmental fields are integral with one another. A closed system model of the universe is contradicted. Such concepts as equilibrium, adaptation, homeostasis, and steady state are outdated.

A *universe of open systems* is a concept that has been increasingly appearing in the literature over the last 20 or 30 years. At the turn of the century, of course, physicists thought they knew all there was to know about the physical worlds. But then, Einstein discovered relativity and Max Planck, quantum theory and Heisenberg, the principle of uncertainty, all of which contradicted Newton, who had dealt with absolutism. The idea of open systems has created a great stir among a lot of people, particularly those scholars in the physical sciences. In the 1920s, Selye was beginning to work with adaptation syndromes; then, in the 1930s, von Bertalanffy proposed negative entropy, but he still fostered the idea of the universe eventually running down. By the 1960s although there were physiologists who were changing the term homeostasis (which means like static) to homeokinesis (which means like motion), people began to note that a universe of open systems was real and that space exploration confirmed the obsolescence of ideas like steady state, homeostasis, adaptation, and equilibrium. Now, in the 1980s, causality is invalid. Bertrand Russell (1958) called it a relic of a bygone age, surviving, like the monarchy, only because it is erroneously supposed to do no harm.

Pattern identifies energy fields. It is the distinguishing characteristic of a field and is perceived of as a single wave. The nature of the pattern changes continuously and innovatively. Each human field pattern is unique and is integral with its own unique environmental field.

Four-dimensionality is defined as a nonlinear domain without spatial or temporal attributes. All reality is postulated to be four-dimensional. With this belief the relative nature of change becomes explicit.

Definitions of human and environmental fields give specificity to the emerging conceptual system. The unitary human being (human field) is defined as an irreducible, four-dimensional energy field identified by pattern and manifesting characteristics different from those of the parts and which cannot be predicted from knowledge of the parts. The environmental field is defined as an irreducible, four-dimensional energy field identified by pattern and manifesting characteristics different from those of the parts. Each environmental field is specific to its given human field. Both change continuously and creatively.

Principles of the Science of Unitary Human Beings

Principles and theories derive from the conceptual system described above. The principles of homeodynamics postulate the nature and direction of change and are stated below.

	Principles of Homeodynamics
Principle of Resonancy	The continuous change from lower to higher frequency wave patterns in human and environmental fields
Principles of Helicy	The continuous, innovative, probabilistic increasing diversity of human and environmental field patterns characterized by non-repeating rhythmicities
Principle of Integrality (formerly titled Principle of Complementarity)	The continuous mutual human field and environmental field process

Theories Derived from the Science of Unitary Human Beings

A theory of accelerating evolution deriving from this conceptual system puts in different perspective today's rapidly changing norms in blood pressure levels, children's behavior, longer waking periods, and other events. Higher frequency wave patterns of growing diversity that portend new norms coordinate with accelerating change. Labels of pathology based on old norms generate hypochondriasis and iatrogenesis. Normal means average. Normal (average) blood pressure readings in all age groups are notably higher today than they were a few decades ago. Evidence that these norms are jeopardizing the public health are insubstantial. Not only has the average waking period lengthened, but sleep/wake continuities are increasingly diverse. Developmental norms have changed significantly in recent years. Gifted children and the so-called hyperactive not uncommonly manifest similar behaviors. It would seem more reasonable to hypothesize hyperactivity as accelerating evolution than to denigrate rhythmicities that diverge from outdated norms and erroneous expectations.

Manifestations of a speeding up of human field rhythms are coordinate with higher frequency environmental field patterns. Radiating increments of widely diverse frequencies are common household accompaniments of everyday life. Atmospheric and cosmological complexity grow. Environmental motion has quickened.

A very high speed transit tube craft that can whisk people across the country by electromagnetic waves at approximately 14,000 miles per hour is already within human capability. Human and environmental fields evolve together. The doomsayers who claim that people are destroying themselves are in error. On the contrary, there is population explosion, increased longevity, escalating levels of science and technology, the development of space communities and multiple other evidences of human developmental potentials in the process of actualization.

With increased longevity, there are growing numbers of older persons. Contrary to a static view engendered by a closed system model of the universe that postulates aging to be a decline, the science of unitary human beings postulates aging to be part of a developmental process; it is continuous from conception through the dying process. Field patterns become increasingly diverse and creative. The aged need less sleep and sleep/wake frequencies become more varied. Higher frequency patterns give meaning to multiple reports of time perceived as racing.

The four-dimensional nature of reality is of further relevance. A nonlinear domain points up the invalidity of chronological age as a basis for differentiating development. In fact, as developmental diversity continues to accelerate, the range and variety of differences between individuals also increases. The more diverse field patterns evolve more rapidly than the less diverse ones. Populations defy so-called normal curves as individual differences multiply.

The emergence of paranormal phenomena as valid subjects for serious scientific research has nonetheless been handicapped by a paucity of viable theories to explain these events. The nature of the paradigm presented here provides a framework for such theories. Four-dimensional reality as conceptualized is a factor in deriving testable hypotheses. The implications for creative health services are notable. Alternative forms of healing are increasingly popular, and some are surprisingly effective. Meditative modalities bespeak "beyond waking" manifestation, and therapeutic touch has been documented as efficacious.

Research findings support the nature of change postulated in the principles of homeodynamics. Investigations into the nature of field patterning with its continuously changing manifestations are underway. The search for indices of patterning has begun. Unitary human field attributes are field manifestations. New tools of measurement are necessary adjuncts to studying questions arising out of a worldview that is different from the prevalent view.

Nursing is concerned with the dying as well as with the living. Unitary human rhythms find expression in the rhythmicity of the living/dying process. Just as aging is deemed developmental, so too is dying hypothesized as developmental. The nature of the dying process and after-death phenomena have gained considerable public and professional interest in recent years, yet rejection of the dying person is all too common. Questionable practices in securing organs for transplantation have led to legislative actions. The concept of one's right-to-die with dignity is being written into people's final testaments. Concomitantly, reports of near-death and after-death experiences are popular reading. The dying process can be studied effectively within this system. The continuity of field patterning after death would seem to be a much more difficult area to investigate, although it is by no means impossible.

The potentialities of this paradigm are several. It is logically and scientifically tenable; it is flexible and open ended; it is researchable. The practical implications for human health and welfare are already demonstrable.

Seeing the world from this viewpoint requires a new synthesis, a creative leap and the inculcation of new attitudes and values. Guiding principles are broad generalizations that require imaginative and innovative modalities for their implementation. A science of unitary human beings identifies nursing's uniqueness and signifies the potential of nurses to fulfill their social responsibility in human service.

REFERENCES

Capra, F. (1982). *The turning point.* New York: Simon and Schuster.

Rogers, M. E. (1970). *An introduction to the theoretical basis of nursing.* Philadelphia: F. A. Davis Co.

Rogers, M. E. (1980). Nursing: A science of unitary man. *In* Riehl, J. P. and Roy, C., eds. *Conceptual models for nursing practice.* New York: Appleton-Century-Crofts.

Russell, B. (1958). *The ABCs of relativity.* New York: New American Library.

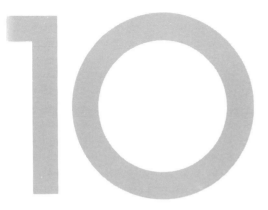

A Critique of Rogers's Framework

ANN L. WHALL

The critique is limited to the two major presentations of Rogers's conceptual system, *An Introduction to the Theoretical Basis of Nursing* (1970) and *Nursing: A Science of Unitary Man* (1980). Rogers's *Science of Unitary Man* is variously characterized as a conceptual system, model, or framework, terms she uses to describe her work.

Structure

HISTORICAL EVOLUTION

Rogers's work demonstrates a slight evolution from 1970 to 1980. In the 1970 work, Rogers presented the background sources that influenced her thinking as she developed her model. It demon-

147

strates the wide variety of knowledge that has influenced her work. These sources range from prehistoric findings unearthed in various digs around the world, to the philosophical discussions of Darwin and Descartes, to discussions of the field theorists Lewin, Burr, and Northrup (Rogers, 1970). In the 1970 work, this background explication covers roughly one-fourth of the work. Very little of this background discussion was presented in the 1980 work, a single chapter. However, it would be helpful if Rogers would update this material in her forthcoming text, for there have been newer and relevant materials presented in the past 15 years.

The conceptual system presented in the 1970 text changes somewhat in the 1980 work as far as terminology is concerned. No substantive differences, however, are noted. In the 1970 text, for example, the major concepts of the model are presented, along with the assumptions on which the model is based. The major relational statements are also presented. In the 1980 work, the concepts are termed building blocks and are presented succinctly along with the principles that relate the concepts.

The major concepts found in the 1970 work are openness, wholeness, unidirectionality, pattern and organization, and sentience: the characteristics of Man. The major principles found in the work are reciprocity, synchrony, helicy, and resonancy. Major concepts found in the 1980 work are energy field, openness, pattern and organization, and four-dimensionality. The principles of helicy, resonancy, and complementarity are defined. In this work the concepts of unidirectionality of life is implicit throughout the work rather than given an explicit identification. The three principles in the 1980 edition are understood to encompass the four prior principles, that is, complementarity, helicy, and resonancy (which encompasses synchrony and reciprocity). Complementarity, which was added to the list, has recently been changed to "integrality." The relationships represented by the principles of reciprocity and synchrony can be identified in the three present principles. Thus a source of possible confusion was eliminated in the 1980 work.

One final note on the historical evolution of the model. Rogers began the 1970 work with a discussion that Man or people are the proper object of nursing's focus. There was a raging debate in the early 1960s as to what was nursing's proper focus. Thanks in large part to Rogers's work, the controversy was resolved.

PHILOSOPHICAL ASSUMPTIONS

In the 1970 work, the philosophical underpinnings of the framework were explicitly stated:

1. Man is a unified whole possessing his own integrity and manifesting characteristics that are more than and different from the sum of his parts.

2. Man and environment are continuously exchanging matter and energy with one another.

3. The life process evolves irreversibly and unidirectionally along the space/time continuum.

4. Pattern and organization identify Man and reflect his innovative wholeness.

5. Man is characterized by the capacity for abstraction and imagery, language and thought, sensation and motion.

The first four assumptions have relevance for all living systems and Man, whereas the fifth assumption refers to Man alone. The assumptions demonstrate Rogers's holistic, nonparticulate, nonmechanistic view. The assumptions have internal congruence.

PRINCIPLES, CONCEPTS, AND PROPOSITIONS

The concepts and principles of Rogers's (1970, 1980) framework are explicitly stated. The principles described above vary slightly in Rogers's two works. The concepts are explicitly discussed and vary hardly at all. Health is not a well-defined concept, being seen as an expression of the life process, and later as a value judgment. It is seen as a value judgment in that society defines the nature of health and illness. Rogers (1980) noted that values are continuously changing and stated "health and sickness, however defined, are expressions of the process of life" (1970, p. 85). Propositions were not explicitly stated in any of Rogers's work. She formulated what she called a theory of accelerating evolution (1980).

DEFINITION OF MAN

Unitary Man is defined as a four-dimensional, negentropic energy field identified by pattern and organization and manifesting characteristics and behaviors that are "different from those of the parts and which cannot be predicted from knowledge of the parts" (1980, p. 332). Rogers (1970) wrote that "Man and his environment are coextensive with the universe" (p. 53). She acknowledged that "it is not an easy matter to envision a universe of interacting wholes" (p. 53). Man and environment with their coextensiveness (or coextension into space/time), are both open systems, which exist together as a whole. The energy field which is Man and the environmental field are unique; Man participates knowingly, and probabilistically in the process of change of self and environment.

Definition of Health

Health is not well defined, but this is consistent with Rogers's position that it is a variable concept depending on cultural interpretation.

Relationship Between Man and Health

In that health is seen as an expression of the life process, and in essence a value placed upon various states by society, the relationship between Man and health is implied rather than explicit. Health is viewed in some relationship to illness. Rogers has written, "health and sickness, however defined, are expressions of the process of life" (1970, p. 85). An inference that may hold is if Man and environment are coextensive, what society calls health and illness are related to Man's environmental state. Since particulate Man is not consistent with unitary Man it would not be consistent with the model to state, for example, that mental health is related to physical health and illness and vice versa. Likewise, it would not be consistent with the model to state that multiple factors "cause" a given illness. Rather, what is seen by society as dichotomous notions, that is, health and illness, are seen by Rogers as expressions of the life process of Man, coextensive with environment. Rogers declined to give health a specific definition because it is value laden and defined differently in each culture. Rogers's works focus on unitary Man. Her description of Man is consistent in that the assumptions regarding Man are internally congruent and the assumptions are congruent with the principles. The notion of health as an expression of life process is consistent with the view of Man. This gives evidence of a sound structure.

Process

Correspondence
Established Knowledge of Man and Health

Man appears to be understood in most other nursing models as the sum of the parts. Rogers wrote of Man as more than the sum of the parts. In this view, Man cannot be predicted from knowledge of the various parts. Most of the other nursing models, however, describe Man as a bio-psycho-social being. This description in Rogers's view is interpreted as a focus on parts rather than on the whole. In essence Rogers focused only on the whole of Man, defined the term as an energy field coextensive with the environment. Therefore, in Rogers's model the understanding of Man is not consistent with other nursing models that discuss Man as greater than the sum of the parts. Parse (1981), who synthesized assumptions from Rogers and existential-phenomenology agreed with Rogers that Man is more than the sum of the parts. Parse and Rogers have consistently followed this belief throughout descriptions of their works. No other nurse theorist defines Man as an energy field.

The dictionary defines Man as "a human being, whether male or female; a member of the human race." In that Rogers used the term Man to refer to either gender, this would be consistent with the dictionary definition of Man. Many other nursing models use the term "person," which in their view eliminates any sexist connotation, but "person" is a concept at a lower level of discourse than required in a theory. Rogers's terminology is different from terminology in the other nursing models. It specifies unitary Man as the science of nursing.

The various definitions of health have been examined by Smith (1983). In general, she found four major understandings of the term: the ability to perform roles, the absence of disease, adaptation, and "the condition of complete development of the individual's potential" (p. 87). Though Rogers declined to define health, she referred to it along with illness and sickness and also discussed health as an expression of the life process, somewhat congruent with Smith's (1983) fourth major definition of the term. There appears to be some inconsistency in that Rogers left the definition of health up to society to define. The concept of health has not been articulated clearly in the Rogers model.

Interrelation of Concepts at the Same Level of Discourse

The four concepts that Rogers uses are broad, in the sense of being all-inclusive, and abstract. Four-dimensionality, for example, is present if you are in space, on earth, and in hospital settings, or in the community. All of the concepts also have a high degree of abstraction, or are separated at great distance from material objects and events. It is difficult to "see" four-dimensionality or to observe coextensive energy fields. All of the concepts are written in abstract terms and are thus at a consistent level of discourse.

With regard to describing and explaining phenomena, Rogers's model has great explanatory power. By using her conceptualizations, one is able to explain multiple phenomena. In the terms of prediction one can predict the general outcome of events but is hampered with the evaluation of this prediction because of the lack of measurement devices or instruments that are either not developed or are not logically consistent with Rogers's model. The concepts of the framework, then, are at a consistent abstract level of discourse. Description and explanatory efforts are fruitful using the model, and prediction is possible; however, measurement of these predicted outcomes is problematic.

The concepts describe Man and environment and explain their

relationship. The nature of other relationships are also explained, as in the way in which time and space are related. If prediction is taken in a general or broad sense, as in predicting Man will age, prediction is possible within this framework. If prediction is taken in a more specific sense, that is, identifying outcomes of specific "treatments" in a given situation, prediction is less possible. Conceptual frameworks, however, are not generally expected to reach this predictive level of specificity. Theories derived from Rogers's work may reach the level of prediction but Rogers's work is broad and abstract.

Relationship to Paradigmatic Perspectives and Philosophical Assumptions

Paradigm refers to worldview. Parse (1981, 1985) discussed that there are two general paradigms represented in nursing conceptual models, the totality and simultaneity paradigms. In the totality worldview (Parse and others, 1985), Man is viewed as a biopsycho-social being, or the totality of these aspects of Man. In the simultaneity view, Man is seen as mutually living and evolving with the environment. The focus on the simultaneity paradigm is thus on the mutual simultaneous interaction of Man with the environment in the life process rather than the various components of Man. In the totality worldview, life processes are described as analogous to a machine. In this view Man is described as separate from environment and a focus is on the parts interacting in a causal manner; entropy and closed boundaries are assumed. In the simultaneity worldview, life processes are viewed as a whole, the focus is upon nonpredictable, noncausal interactions of Man and environment. Negentropy and open, nonbounded systems are assumed. From this description, it is clear that Rogers's approach represents a simultaneity worldview. Her focus is definitely on the whole and not upon causality, boundaries, or separation.

In this framework the concepts are related to the principles and the principles to the assumptions. In other words, there is a close integration of all these features of the framework. For example, the principle of helicy states that (1970, p. 101), "helicy is a function of continuous innovative change growing out of the mutual interaction of Man and environment along a spiralling longitudinal axis bound in space-time." The third assumption states that (1970, p. 50), "the life process evolves irreversibly and unidirectionally along the space-time continuum." The building block, four-dimensionality describes in part an open human and environmental field not bound by space and time. In other words, Man is conceived of as an open system evolving irreversibly and unidirectionally in a spiralling longitudinal axis across space and time. Man is an open system moving with environment through this unidirectional journey through spacetime. The concepts, principles, and assumptions are all interrelated and are thus logically consistent or correspondent with each other.

Description and Meaning of Principles, Concepts, and Propositions

The principles are closely interwoven with each other as are the concepts and assumptions. All of these theoretical elements are logically interrelated or consistent with each other. Thus, with only three principles, a few major concepts and five assumptions, Rogers has explained the nature of Man and life process. The elements are so abstract that they are able to encompass all situations which makes the framework universally applicable. Much work, however, must be done by nurse researchers and nurses in practice to bring the relationships and concepts to a less abstract level for testing.

Rogers's framework is somewhat hard to understand. For example, four-dimensionality cannot be fully explained because of the lack of adequate terminology. The framework is therefore deep in meaning but not necessarily beyond the grasp of ordinary minds. The language of a theory is at a high level of abstraction, which leads to the possibility of inferring regarding life situations. It leads scholars beyond where they are and offers researchers an opportunity to bring the concepts to another level of discourse for testing. The terms Rogers used are not found in the dictionary; these terms describe new and uncharted relationships. In this sense, her work has led to new understandings of nursing science. While some of the language is new and the framework is written at an abstract level, Rogers defined clearly her principles, concepts, and the structure of the relationship among same. Rogers did not reverse herself or give a definition of a concept and then use the concept to infer contrary things or situations. However, the concept "four dimensionality" is defined primarily in a negative sense, statements are made about what it is not, almost more than what it is. There is an incompleteness to the discussion that limits clarity of meaning. To the extent that incomplete descriptions are unclear, there is a certain lack of clarity in this regard. Also measurement indices for the concepts lack clarity.

On the other hand, one may argue that the theorist does not need to do all of the explication; this can and should be done by researchers and those who test the framework in practice.

COHERENCE

Relation of Framework to other Theories

Although Rogers's framework may not appear to be directly related to most other nursing models, when other models are based on open systems, there are certain similarities between Rogers's model and certain views expressed within these other nursing models. There are at least two other models either closely related to or based upon Rogers's model—the Newman (1979) and Parse (1981) models. Newman grounded her views of health as expanded consciousness in Rogers's principles and Parse synthesized Rogers's framework with tenets from existential phenomenology to create the assumptions of her theory. Several other nurse theorists speak of open systems but do not consistently demonstrate the same definition throughout their work.

Terms used by Rogers, such as energy field, helicy, and four-dimensionality, are not found in other nursing models, although certain relationships represented in other models are congruent with aspects of Rogers's framework.

Logical Flow from Assumptions to Propositions

As discussed above a logical flow is clearly evident in Rogers's model. A universe of open systems is presented at the outset and the concept of openness is further described in the principles of helicy and complementarity. There is no inconsistency between any portions of the framework. All elements are consistent with each other and in a sense flow from each other.

Kaplan discussed norms of coherence (1964, p. 314), as in part the need for theory to fit with the body of knowledge that has been established by various methods. He discussed telepathy as a new notion not yet having the "click of relation." Telepathy was something, although not well described until recently, that almost everyone knew existed. Many of Rogers's statements have this "click of relation" and although not explicated in existing knowledge, may express something known intuitively. The "click of relation" has been used to criticize the contribution of Rogers's framework. Some people say, "We already knew that." Kaplan (1964) said that theories are examined for their contribution not just on axiomatic or logical principles, but also in terms of other existing evidence. The "click of relation" is one type of evidence.

Symmetry and Aesthetics

In that Rogers has explained the nature of Man, and life process in four concepts, three principles, and five assumptions, her framework has simplicity. It appears to have balance and clarity in that each idea is defined succinctly and remains consistent throughout her work. The beauty lies in the simplicity and balance. Rogers's framework is symmetrical and aesthetic.

PRAGMATICS

Use of Framework in Practice and Research

There are many examples in the literature and in Rogers's (1970) textbook that purport to be an explication in research related to a portion of her framework. A critical issue that has surfaced in the past few years is that several of these attempts have purportedly been identified by Rogers and others as inconsistent with the framework. Some research studies supposedly testing Rogers's model are cause and effect relationship studies. There is no clear published evidence of the testing of Rogers's noncausal framework in research.

There are, however, multiple research studies that purport to support the framework. These studies and approaches are named in discussions of Rogers's model (Fitzpatrick and Whall, 1983). The issues with all studies is not their purported support for the framework, but rather if the conceptualization and methodology are logically consistent with Rogers's model both in terms of theory and operationalization. As discussed above, there is controversy in this area. That important point aside, in general one may state that support for the framework in terms of research has been reported. It is clear that the abstract level of the framework leads to a plethora of research questions that could be and are posed. Because of the level of abstraction, however, there are often questions raised as to how one might measure certain concepts and relationships. The measurement issue both in terms of operational definitions and instrumentation is at a critical juncture. Researchers will undoubtedly continue their quest for these necessities, but comprehensive, in-depth discussions of the ways in which one may validly address these issues is greatly needed.

In both the 1970 and 1980 texts, general guidelines are offered for practice. In addition, Rogers has offered suggestions for practice both in oral presentations and in other works. These practice suggestions have been most helpful, but too general in nature to demonstrate the specificity necessary to guide practice. Published critiques with clear explanations of the issues involved would encourage "moves down the ladder" to testing in research and practice.

Generally, the theorist is not expected to do this work alone, but assistance in this regard both from Rogers and others is needed. There appears to be a reluctancy on the part of some to attempt a "move down the ladder." Their reluctance is due in part to the lack of guidelines for this effort.

Contribution of Nursing Science

Kaplan (1964) stated that from the "vulgar" issues of practicality, the question is, what can the theory do for science? (p. 319). In this view, scientific formulation should not just be judged on the basis of practicality alone. Kaplan argued that a publication that stirs thought, debate, and argument may well contribute more to science than one that is found very practical. If a theory guides and stimulates scientific inquiry, it is in this view judged as making a very important scientific contribution. Thus the value of the theory "lies not only in the answers it gives but in the new questions it raises" (p. 320). Theories that explain disparate views thus contribute greatly to science; however, those that encourage roaring debates, although later rejected, also contribute to science. The sharing of ideas, questions, and techniques related to theory advance science greatly.

On all of these counts, Rogers's theoretical framework has contributed to nursing science. It has generated lively debates and seems to have raised more questions that it answers. It has explained disparate views while engendering debate regarding techniques that may be used to measure concepts and relationships. The debates engendered by her model have in a sense forced nursing to move on. In a sense, it forced nurse scholars to question and seek answers again and again. If this, as Kaplan has stated, is in essence the value of a theory, Rogers's framework will stand as a milestone. This accomplishment, Kaplan has written, will hold, regardless of the final state of rejection or acceptance of the theory.

REFERENCES

Fitzpatrick, J., and Whall, A. eds. (1983). *Conceptual models of nursing: Analysis and application*. Bowie, MD: Brady Communications.

Kaplan, A. (1964). *The conduct of inquiry*. Scranton: Chandler Publishing Co.

Newman, M. (1979). *Theory development in nursing*. Philadelphia: F. A. Davis Co.

Parse, R. R. (1981). *Man-living-health: A theory of nursing*. New York: John Wiley & Sons.

Parse R. R., Coyne, A. B., and Smith, M. J. (1985). *Nursing research: Qualitative methods*. Bowie, MD: Brady Communications.

Rogers, M. E. (1970). *An introduction to the theoretical basis of nursing*. Philadelphia: F. A. Davis Co.

Rogers, M. E. (1980). Nursing: A science of unitary man. *In* J. Riehl and C. Roy, eds., *Conceptual models for nursing practice*. New York: Appleton-Century-Crofts.

11

Man-Living-Health Theory of Nursing

ROSEMARIE RIZZO PARSE

EDITORIAL PERSPECTIVE

Parse (1981, 1985) describes Man as an open being free to choose meaning in situation. She believes Man reveals and conceals values in transforming to what is not yet. Man co-creates patterns of relating in interchange with the environment. Man structures meaning multidimensionally in cocreating rhythmical patterns while cotranscending with the possibles. This view is consistent with the simultaneity paradigm. Consistent with Rogers, Parse (1981) wrote of health as a process of becoming. She further specified health as lived value priorities, a nonlinear entity that cannot be qualified as good, bad, more, or less. Parse (1981) differs from Rogers (1970, 1980) in that she does not view Man as an energy field, but rather as an open being who cocreates personal health. Parse (1981) also posits multidimen-

159

sionality rather than four-dimensionality as the various universes
Man lives all at once. The language in the works of Rogers (1970,
1980) and Parse (1981) clearly designates nursing science as
distinct from other sciences.

In the following chapter, Parse specifies the principles,
concepts, and theoretical structures of the theory of Man-Living-Health and discusses the research and practice methodologies.

As discussed earlier in this book, in the scientific discipline of
nursing, there are at least two equally important and valuable extant paradigms, the totality paradigm and the simultaneity paradigm (Parse and others, 1985). These paradigms are distinguished
by worldviews of Man and Health, the two phenomena with which
nursing concerns itself. Man-Living-Health is a theory evolving from
the simultaneity paradigm. This theory is based on the belief that
Man is an open being, more than and different from the sum of
parts in mutual simultaneous interchange with the environment who
chooses from options and bears responsibility for choices. Man cocreates patterns of relating with the environment and is recognized
by these patterns. Health is viewed as a process of becoming experienced by the individual. Health is Man's unfolding. It is Man's
lived experiences, a nonlinear entity that cannot be qualified by
terms such as good, bad, more, or less (Parse, 1981). It is not Man
adapting or coping. Unitary Man's health is a synthesis of values,
a way of living. It is not the opposite of disease or a state that man
has, but rather is a continuously changing process that Man cocreates (Parse, 1981).

It is from these general beliefs that the Man-Living-Health theory emerges. This is a unitary phenomenon that refers to man's
becoming through cocreating rhythmical patterns in open interchange with the environment. In order to focus on the essential
nature of process in this theory, *ing* ending words, or participles,
are used throughout the description of the theory. This is to make
specific the idea of Man's living of health as an ever-changing process. The hyphens connecting these words make Man-Living-Health
a construct unto itself. The unity of Man-Living-Health is the focus

of the nursing theory, thus there is no reference in the theory to Man as the sum of parts with biological, social, psychological, and spiritual attributes. This does not mean that these attributes are negated, but rather that they are viewed within the context of Man's wholeness as shown through profiles and qualities.

Philosophical Assumptions

The assumptions, written at the philosophical level of discourse, of Man-Living-Health emerge from a combination of Rogers's principles of helicy, complementarity (now called integrality), and resonancy, plus the four building blocks of energy field, pattern and organization, openness, and four-dimensionality (Rogers, 1970, 1980) with the tenets of human subjectivity and intentionality and the concepts of coconstitution, coexistence, and situated freedom from existential phenomenological thought. This combination created the synthesis of the nine assumptions underpinning the theory of Man-Living-Health (Parse, 1981, p. 36), which have been further synthesized into the following three assumptions:

Assumption 1.
MAN-LIVING-HEALTH IS FREELY CHOOSING PERSONAL MEANING IN SITUATIONS IN THE INTERSUBJECTIVE PROCESS OF RELATING VALUE PRIORITIES.

This means that Man-Living-Health is Man through subject-to-subject-interchange in situation assigns meaning which reflects personal values. Values are shown in the choice of meaning that Man gives to a situation. For example, several persons can experience a moment in time together, such as attending the same event, yet the experience for each person is different. Each chooses the meaning given to the event from personal value priorities.

Assumption 2.
MAN LIVING-HEALTH IS COCREATING RHYTHMICAL PATTERNS OF RELATING IN OPEN INTERCHANGE WITH THE ENVIRONMENT.

This means that Man-Living-Health is Man and environment interrelating in a way that the evolving patterns distinguish one from another. The prefix "co" means "together with"; thus Man together with environment creates the pattern of each. Man is distinguishable as Man and environment as environment, yet each is a coparticipant in the creation of the other.

Assumption 3.
MAN-LIVING-HEALTH IS COTRANSCENDING MULTIDIMENSIONALLY WITH THE UNFOLDING POSSIBLES.

This means that Man-Living-Health is Man moving beyond self at all levels of the universe as dreams become actualities. Cotranscending means moving beyond with others and the environment multidimensionally. Multidimensionally refers to the various levels of the universe that Man experiences all at once. Specifically the term refers to explicit-tacit knowing. Not all choices are made from the explicit level. Man chooses possiblities from the whole sense of the situation. With each situation there are multiple possibles unfolding. What unfolds surfaces in relationship to others and the environment as dreams of what can be become actualities.

The assumptions express in philosophical terms the beliefs that underpin the theory of Man-Living-Health. The most significant distinction of this theory from other theories is the belief that Man, more than and different from the sum of the parts, evolves mutually with the environment, participates in cocreating personal health by choosing meanings in situations, and conveys meanings that are personal values reflecting dreams and hopes.

Principles of Man-Living-Health

Three major themes emerge from these philosophical assumptions: meaning, rhythmicity, and cotranscendence. Each leads to a principle of Man-Living-Health. The principles, written at the theoretical level of discourse, are:

Structuring meaning multidimensionally is cocreating reality through the languaging of valuing and imaging. The essential concepts of this principle are imaging, valuing and languaging. (Parse, 1981, p. 42)

Cocreating rhythmical patterns of relating is living the paradoxical unity of revealing-concealing, enabling-limiting while connecting-separating. The essential concepts are revealing-concealing, enabling-limiting, and connecting-separating. (Parse, 1981, p. 50)

Cotranscending with the possibles is powering unique ways of originating in the process of transforming. The essential concepts of this principle are powering, originating and transforming. (Parse, 1981, p. 55)

Principle 1.
STRUCTURING MEANING MULTIDIMENSIONALLY IS COCREATING REALITY THROUGH THE LANGUAGING OF VALUING AND IMAGING.

This principle, structuring meaning multidimensionally, interrelates the concepts of imaging, valuing, and languaging. Structuring meaning multidimensionally evolves from the assumptions and means that Man constructs meaning from many levels of the universe, from the tacit and explicit, in the cocreating of what is real. Languaging reflects images and values through speaking and moving. Health is an expression of values at the moment, the meaning given to a situation.

There are two kinds of meaning: ultimate meaning, Man's conceptualization of purpose in life, and the meaning moments of everyday life. The latter confronts Man in daily living. Both kinds change through the living of new experiences (Parse, and others, 1985). Every day as one lives new experiences, meaning boundaries are pushed forward; there is a stretching of the meaning moment beyond what it is. As one begins to relate new meanings to daily events, ultimate meaning changes. With each everyday experience, Man structures the meaning that shapes personal knowledge, explicitly-tacitly, all at once.

Imaging is the picturing or making real of events, ideas, and people. Valuing is the living of cherished beliefs. The cherished beliefs are shown through languaging by speaking and moving, which is the way one represents the structure of personal reality.

Principle 2.
COCREATING RHYTHMICAL PATTERNS OF RELATING IS LIVING THE PARADOXICAL UNITY OF REVEALING-CONCEALING, ENABLING-LIMITING, WHILE CONNECTING-SEPARATING.

This principle interrelates the concepts of revealing-concealing, enabling-limiting, and connecting-separating and evolves from the assumptions.

Man and environment cocreate a rhythmical interchange. Connecting-separating is the rhythmical process of distancing and relating, that is, moving in one direction and away from others, yet always toward greater diversity. Connecting-separating with others and projects is enabling-limiting. Every time one makes a choice, there are an infinite number of possibilities within that choice and also an infinite number of limitations. In the rhythmical patterns of relating with others, one is revealing-concealing the who one is. One cannot tell all there is about self to self or to others. All is not known explicitly; Man is always unfolding mystery. There is always the known in the unknown and the unknown in the known. Man cocreates patterns with others and the environment, and there are an infinite number of possibilities and limitations in any choice. One reveals and conceals self in each situation.

Principle 3.
COTRANSCENDING WITH THE POSSIBLES IS POWERING UNIQUE WAYS OF ORIGINATING IN THE PROCESS OF TRANSFORMING.

This principle interrelates the concepts of powering, originating, and transforming, and evolves from the assumptions. Man is always changing, always in the process of transforming. The changing is moving beyond where one is to the not yet. Changing, moving beyond, is sparked by an energizing force, powering originating. Originating means creating anew; it is generating unique ways of living. Unique ways of living surface in Man's continual interrogation of relationships and connections with people and projects. The connections are not unusual but the way the connections are lived show the uniqueness. One is unique in that one is irreplaceable—in close relationships and creative projects.

Powering is the energizing force in originating. It is Man's nature to power. According to Tillich (1952), to be is the power to exist. Powering is the pushing-resisting of interhuman encounters that originates the uniqueness in the process of transforming. Transforming is the changing of change (Parse, 1981). Change itself is a continuous ongoing process in the Man-environment interrelationship. It is recognized by increasing diversity: the ways a pattern is both the same and different all at once. Transforming occurs through struggling and moving beyond. It unfolds as the familiar is seen in a different light, thus shifting the view and illuminating new possibles.

The three principles of Man-Living-Health, then, specify the theory and flow directly from the philosophical assumptions. There are nine major concepts in the theory; three from each of the principles. The concepts are imaging, valuing, languaging, revealing-concealing, enabling-limiting, connecting-separating, powering, originating, and transforming. In creating propositions from principles, it is appropriate to use one concept from each of the three principles.

Theoretical Structures

The theoretical structures of Man-Living-Health are nondirectional propositions. Nondirectional propositions are noncausal in nature and consistent with the assumptions and principles. The theoretical structures are written at the theoretical level and are designed to guide practice and research. To make these operational in practice and research, practice propositions must be derived and lived experiences chosen for study. The three theoretical published structures are: (1) powering is a way of revealing-concealing imaging, (2) originating is a manifestation of enabling-limiting valuing, and (3) transforming unfolds in the languaging of connecting-separating (Parse, 1981, p. 72). Others may be derived.

Research and Practice Traditions in Nursing

The research and practice methodologies utilized in the discipline of nursing are borrowed from other disciplines. Nursing does not have research and practice traditions of its own. Quantitative and qualitative methods of research used to enhance nursing science presently flow from the natural sciences and from the human sciences, respectively. The nursing process, the only practice methodology in nursing, evolves from the discipline of philosophy and does not flow from an ontological base in the discipline of nursing. The steps of assessing, planning, implementing, and evaluating— the steps of the problem-solving process—are not unique to nursing. The nursing process does not evolve from the science of nursing. The next step in the evolutionary process of nursing as a discipline is to identify research and practice methodologies that flow from from the ontological base of nursing. The practice of nursing evolving from a theory must logically connect to that theory. Practice is the empirical life of the theory, which means that the practice of one theory would be very different from the practice of another. In any discipline then, there are many theories and thus many practice and research methodologies. Theorists and other scholars have the task of honing the methodologies for prac-

TABLE 11-1
Man-Living-Health Practice Methodology

Dimensions
- Illuminating meaning is shedding light through uncovering the what was, is, and will be, as it is appearing now; it happens in *explicating what is*
- Synchronizing rhythms happens in *dwelling with* the pitch, yaw, and roll of the interhuman cadence
- Mobilizing transcendence happens in *moving beyond* the meaning moment to what is not-yet

Processes
- Explicating is making clear what is appearing now through languaging
- Dwelling with is giving self over to the flow of the struggle in connecting-separating
- Moving beyond is propelling toward the possibles in transforming

tice and research peculiar to the belief system on which their own theory is based.

Man-Living-Health Practice Methodology

The goal in the practice methodology of the theory of Man-Living-Health is in the quality of life as perceived by the person and the family. The contextual situations are nurse-person or nurse-group participation. In the practice methodology of Man-Living-Health, there are dimensions and processes (see Table 11-1). The dimensions are illuminating meaning, synchronizing rhythms, and mobilizing transcendence. The processes are empirical activities: explicating, dwelling with, and moving beyond. The dimensions and processes flow directly from the principles that flow from the assumptions of the Man-Living-Health theory. There is a clear connection, then, between the practice methodology and the theory itself. For example, illuminating meaning through explicating comes directly from the first principle, structuring meaning multidimensionally. Synchronizing rhythms through dwelling with the ebb and flow of human encounters evolves directly from the second principle, cocreating rhythmical patterns. Mobilizing transcendence through moving beyond evolves directly from the third principle, cotranscending with the possibles.

DIMENSIONS AND PROCESSES IN THE PRACTICE OF MAN-LIVING-HEALTH

Illuminating Meaning

Illuminating meaning involves shedding light through the uncovering of what was, and will be as it is appearing now. Through explicating what is at this moment simply joins what was and what will be. One is only in the moment, which is fleeting. The nurse guides individuals and families to relate the meaning of the situation. In telling about the meaning, persons share thoughts and feelings with one another, which in itself changes the meaning of a situation by making it more explicit.

Synchronizing Rhythms

Synchronizing rhythms happens in dwelling with the pitch, yaw, and roll of the interhuman cadence—the turning, spinning, and thrusting of human relationships. Pitch, yaw, and roll represent the ups and downs, the struggles, the moments of joy, the unevenness of day-to-day living. The nurse with the Man-Living-Health belief system does not try to calm these rhythms, or try to balance or help the family adapt, but rather the nurse goes with the rhythm set by the family. The nurse moves with the flow of the rhythm, stays with the family's views, leading the family through discussion to recognize the harmony that exists within its own lived context. There is always a way to find the harmony in what appears to be the conflict in the spinning and turning of human relationships. This way of practicing nursing represents a departure from the traditional. It is grounded in a different belief system. Commonly used "techniques" in nursing do not fit with the Man-Living-Health theory. For example, reality therapy does not fit with the Man-Living-Health theory. The nurse practicing the principles of Man-Living-Health would go with the person in what appears to be confusion and lead the person to uncover the personal meaning of the situation; the nurse focuses on the person's own meaning of that moment. In discussing the situation, the meaning changes for the person and the way the confusion is lived also changes.

Mobilizing Transcendence

Mobilizing transcendence happens through moving beyond the meaning moment to what is not yet. It focuses on dreaming of the possibles and planning to reach for the dreams. The nurse guides individuals and families to plan for the changing of lived health patterns—these patterns uncovered in the illuminating of meaning, synchronizing of rhythms, and mobilizing of transcendence.

The practice of nursing according to the theory of Man-Living-Health is a different kind of nursing. It is not offering professional advice and opinions stemming from the personal value system of the nurse. It is not a canned approach to cure. It is a subject-to-subject-interrelationship, a loving, true presence with the other to promote health and the quality of life.

The specific processes inherent in the dimensions are defined as follows. *Explicating* is a process of making clear what is appearing now through languaging; *Dwelling with* is giving self over to the flow of the struggle in connecting-separating; and *moving beyond* is propelling toward the possibles in transforming (Table 11-1).

The dimensions and processes described above form the practice methodology of Man-Living-Health. It is clear that the practice of the Man-Living-Health is not congruent with the nursing process as used in most of the nursing literature. The nursing process assumes that the health professional is the authority on health and that the person adapts or can be "fixed," which is a belief consistent with the theories in the totality paradigm but is opposed to the belief system of the Man-Living-Health theory.

Theoretical Structures
and Practice Propositions

The theoretical structures with practice propositions below include a general discussion of nursing practice in light of the propositions and the dimensions and processes of practices discussed above. The details of nursing practice can only be specified in the context of particular nurse-person and nurse-group situations—a task beyond the scope of this paper.

The first theoretical structure, *powering is a way of revealing-concealing imaging,* can be stated as *struggling to live goals discloses the significance of the situation.* That is the proposition at a less abstract level and at this level guides practice. The focus of nursing practice is on illuminating the process of revealing-concealing unique ways a person and family can mobilize transcendence in considering new dreams, to image new possibles. In a nurse-family process, members share their thoughts and feelings about a situation, which both tells and does not tell all they know in the continuous struggle to meet personal goals. In disclosing the significance of the situation, the meaning of it changes for the family members, thus for the family.

The second theoretical structure, *originating is a manifestation of enabling-limiting valuing,* can be stated at the next lower level of abstraction as *creating anew shows one's cherished beliefs and leads in a directional movement.* The focus of nursing practice with a person and family is on illuminating ways of being alike and different from others in changing values. In a nurse-family process, by synchronizing rhythms, the members uncover the opportunities and limitations created by the decisions made in choosing irreplaceable ways of being together. The choices of new ways of being together mobilizes transcendence.

For the third theoretical structure, *transforming unfolds in the languaging of connecting-separating,* a practice proposition at the next lower level of abstraction is *changing views emerge in speaking and moving with others.* The focus of nursing practice is on illuminating meaning of relating ways of being together as various changing perspectives shed different light on the familiar, which gives rise to new possibles. In synchronizing rhythms in a nurse-family process, members relate their values through speech and movement; thus views change and through mobilizing transcendence ways of relating change. When changing views are talked about among family members new possibles are seen and thus the ways of relating among family members change.

Nursing practice from the perspective of the Man-Living-Health theory is very different from practice based on other belief systems. It is essential that the practice methodology be congruent with the philosophical assumptions and the theory. This means that each theory of nursing should have a relevant practice methodology evolving from its ontological base.

Research Related to Man-Living-Health

An emerging research methodology for inquiry consistent with the ontological base of Man-Living-Health has been developed and is discussed below. Prior to its development, research related to Man-Living-Health was implemented utilizing the qualitative methods from other human sciences. The book *Nursing Research: Qualitative Methods* (Parse and others 1985) reveals support of Man-Living-Health as a theory, through phenomenological, descriptive, and ethnographic methods. The results of five major studies appear in this work: there is a phenomenological study of *health*, one on *persisting in change*, an exploratory study on the *lived experience of being exposed to toxic chemicals*, an ethnographic study on *aging*, and a case study on *retirement*.

These five studies demonstrate similar findings that complement each other and support the theory of Man-Living-Health. Meaning, rhythmicity, and transcendence, the three major themes that surface from the assumptions and give rise to the three principles of Man-Living-Health, can be seen in varying ways in all studies. For the phenomenological study on health, 400 subjects between the ages of 7 and 90 were invited to describe a situation in which they experienced health. The common elements across all 400 were energy, harmony, and plentitude. These were demonstrated by all four groups, but there was a clear shift in focus from one group to the other. The shift was from an intense focus on movement for the young group to a more contemplative engagement with purposeful projects and activities in the older subjects.

The phenomenological study on *persisting in change* revealed some similarities with the middle-aged group in the health study in that the subjects struggled with the certainty-uncertainty in beginning new projects in light of reordering their interrelationships with others. There was considerable turbulence shown by subjects in the persisting in change study. Immersion in movement and struggle was evident here as it was in the health study.

In the exploratory study related to the meaning of firefighters being exposed to toxic chemicals, the movement and struggle was seen when those who had been exposed deliberately chose to stay in the situation, accepting the risk of the known present danger and future uncertainties. For these individuals, the immersion in this struggle focused on the meaning of their interrelationships and reevaluation of their priorities.

Contemplative engagement with purposefulness and significant completions was most evident in the oldest group of the health study; it coincides both with the results in the ethnographic study and with the results of the retirement study. In the ethnographic study, contemplative engagement was seen in the quiet struggle of the old to make livable the concrete realities of their changing worlds (Parse and others, 1985). In the case study, contemplative engagement was seen as a retired couple struggled with the decision to retire or continue to work, and with their subsequent satisfaction with their retirement. The changing patterns of the couple's life in retirement generated new possibilities, different relationships, a more flexible structure, and more satisfying individual projects.

In all five studies, there was a shifting of the rhythms in connecting-separating as the subjects created unique ways of transforming life patterns in light of changing value priorities. This conclusion gives evidence of the support for the Man-Living-Health theory using methods from the human sciences.

Man-Living-Health Research Methodology

In building the research methodology for the Man-Living-Health theory, three major essentials were considered: (1) the basic assumptions of Man-Living-Health (described above); (2) the principles of Man-Living-Health (described above); and (3) the principles of methodology construction derived from Kaplan (1964) and Sondheim (1984) described below.

Methodology is the description, the explanation, and the justification of methods; the methodology encompasses the techniques and principles of methods (Kaplan, 1964). Methods are the general techniques and philosophical principles relating to the science. They include formulating concepts, building models and theories, and providing explanations (Kaplan 1964). There is an art to the development of a methodology. The art of making science, just as the art of making art, requires order, design, composition, balance, and harmony (Sondheim, 1984). Order is a sequenced arrangement. Design is a blueprint that reveals an overall pattern. Composition is a blending in the creation of an integral whole. Balance is symmetry, an aesthetic simplicity, and harmony is the congruence of the constituent elements. The methodology, then, is ordered in a particular arrangement following a design composed of a blending of ideas. The methodology is symmetrical in structure and congruent in substance. These principles of methodology construction synthesized from Kaplan's (1964) and Sondheim's (1984) works are:

- The methodology is constructed to be in harmony with and evolve from the ontological beliefs of the research tradition.
- The methodology is an overall design of precise processes that adhere to scientific rigor.
- The methodology specifies the order within the processes appropriate for inquiry within the research tradition.
- The methodology is an aesthetic composition with balance in form.

A research tradition includes both ontological and methodological elements; the ontology is the belief system about the phenomena of concern in a discipline (in this case the theory of Man-Living-Health) and the methodology is the approach to inquiry (as set forth below).

The methodology derived for the Man-Living-Health theory includes: (1) identification of major entities for study, (2) scientific processes of investigation; and (3) details of the processes appropriate for inquiry. (Table 11-2).

Entities For Study

The major entities from the ontology to be considered for inquiry are lived experiences. Two aspects of lived experiences to be

TABLE 11-2
Man-Living-Health Research Methodology

I. Entities for Study: Lived experiences
  A. Common human experiences surfacing in the Man-environment interrelationship
  B. Health-related experiences reflecting
    1. Being-becoming
    2. Value priorities
    3. Negentropic unfolding
    4. Quality of life
II. Processes of the Method
  A. Participant Selection
  B. Dialogical Engagement
  C. Extraction-Synthesis (dwelling with)
    1. Extract essences from transcribed description (participant's language)
    2. Synthesize essences (researcher's language)
    3. Formulate a proposition from each participant's synthesized essences
    4. Extract concepts from the formulated propositions of all participants
    5. Synthesis a structure of the lived experience from the extracted concepts
  D. Heuristic Interpretation
    1. Structural integration
    2. Conceptual interpretation

considered in selecting the entity for study are nature and structure. The nature of lived experiences are that they are common human experiences surfacing in the Man-environment interrelationship; and that they are health-related experiences, reflecting: being-becoming, value priorities, negentropic unfolding, and quality of life.

The lived experience studied, then, is one whose nature is consistent with these specifics. For example, the lived experience is a universal experience such as "waiting," not an experience like "undergoing heart transplant." Waiting is a common human experience surfacing from the Man-environment interrelationship. It is health-related in that it is a chosen way of being with a situation, thus a value priority and an essence of becoming. "Undergoing heart transplant" is not a common human experience, nor is it a way of being. Sometimes one aspect of a lived experience is studied like "feeling restricted" or "feeling hopeful." These aspects are one side of the paradoxical rhythm. Both sides of the rhythm surface in descriptions of lived experiences, but ordinarily one's lived experiences do not present themselves explicitly as "feeling restricted-feeling free" or "feeling hopeful-feeling hopeless." One aspect is usually fore and the other ground, yet both are inextricably present.

Structure is the paradoxical living of the remembered, the now moment and the not-yet all at once. This is uncovered through the dialogical engagement in the Man-Living-Health research method. The entity, the lived experience, the particular nature of which is outlined above, is investigated to uncover its structure as lived by the participants.

The research interrogatory is a statement demonstrating the seeking of understanding. For example, a research question is, What is the structure of the lived experience of waiting? The researcher embarks on a study then, to uncover the structure of lived experiences. Experiences are lived in multidimensional universes, all at once. An understanding of an entity can be gained through the processes of the method.

PROCESSES OF THE METHOD

The processes of the method include participant selection, dialogical engagement, extraction-synthesis, and heuristic interpretation.

Participant Selection

Participant selection is carefully done. Persons are invited to participate who live the experience. An assumption is that a person who agrees to participate in a study about a particular lived experience can give an authentic accounting of that experience when engaged in dialogue with the researcher. Two to ten participants are considered adequate in this method.

Dialogical Engagement

Dialogical engagement is the research-participant discussion. This is an intersubjective "being with," in which researcher and participant live the I-thou process as they move through an unstructured discussion about the lived experience. The I-thou process is one in which the researcher is truly present to the participant in discussion as the remembered, the now and the not-yet unfold all at once.

The researcher comes to the participant after having dwelled with the meaning of the lived experience and after having created some dialogue directional ideas. The dialogue direction emerges from the nature and structure of the lived experience. It is not a rigid set of questions to be asked, but rather, a sense of the ideas to be shared in centering the discussion on the entity as lived by the participants. For example, how the experience came to be, what its presence is now, and what is envisioned. The discussion is tape-recorded, and the dialogue is transcribed to typed format for easy reading for dwelling with the description.

Extraction-Synthesis

Extraction-synthesis occurs through dwelling with the transcribed research-participant dialogue. "Dwelling with" is a way of centering in dialogical engagement with the typed descriptions. The researcher dialogues with the descriptions. Dwelling with permeates the entire extraction-synthesis process. The term extract was chosen to convey the meaning of the essence of a concentrate. The process of moving to incrementally higher levels of abstraction, that is, from the descriptions to the structure, happens through creative conceptualization. And that happens through inventing, which is synthesizing in the researcher's perspective; abstracting, which is moving up the ladder of discourse; and abiding with logic, which is adhering to semantical consistency.

The details of extraction-synthesis include five major processes: (1) Extracting essences from transcribed descriptions (participant's language): an extracted essence is a complete expression of a core idea described by the participant. (2) Synthesizing essences (researcher's language): a synthesized essence is an expression of the core idea of the extracted essence conceptualized by the researcher. (3) Formulating a proposition from each participant's description: a proposition is a nondirectional statement conceptualized by the researcher joining the core idea of the synthesized essences from each participant. (4) Extracting concepts from the formulated propositions of all participants: an extracted concept is the idea that captures the central meaning of the proposition. (5) Synthesizing a structure of the lived experience from the extracted concepts: a synthesized structure is a statement conceptualized by the researcher joining the core concepts. The structure as evolved answers the research questions, what is the structure of this lived experience?

Heuristic Interpretation

Heuristic interpretation includes structural integration and conceptual interpretation. Structural integration is connecting the proposition and the structure to the theory. Conceptual interpretation further specifies the structure of the lived experience with the concepts of Man-Living-Health, leading to a specific theoretical structure from the principles. The findings of the study are in the essences of the propositions. The structure of the lived experience as uncovered through dialogue and extraction-synthesis is interpreted in light of the ontological base, and the structure is discussed and connected to the principles of Man-Living-Health. The heuristic interpretation weaves the ideas of the structure as lived into the theory and propels it beyond to posit ideas for research studies and possible practice activities.

This emerging methodology differs from all other methods. It differs from those in the totality paradigm in that those methods call for a focus on linear causality in the Man-environment interrelationship (Table 11-3). The ontology of the totality paradigm leads to methods of inquiry that seek cause-effect and associative relationships among variables in order to make predictions. The Man-Living-Health research methodology is also different from other qualitative methods (Table 11-4). The areas of difference lie primarily in the way the processes are expressed and in the way they are lived. The key difference is that dialogical engagement is

TABLE 11-3
Differences With Quantitative Research Methods

	Totality Paradigm Methods	Man-Living-Health Method
Conceptual:	Phenomena are attributes of Man reduced to variables for studying cause-effect and associative relationships	Entities for study are lived experiences–common experiences related to health as defined in Man-Living-Health
Methodological	Data collection instruments elicit information from subjects through forced-answer questionnaires or observational techniques	Researcher-participant dialogue elicits descriptions of personal accounts of the participants' lived experiences
	Data analyses reduce data to numerical digits for statistical comparison and inference	Extraction-synthesis moves participants' descriptions through conceptualizations by the researcher to syntheses of structures of lived experiences
Interpretive:	Hypotheses are tested and predictions are made about relationships	Structures of lived experiences are created and theories are enhanced through heuristic interpretation

the way of eliciting a description from the participant of the entity being studied. The extraction-synthesis process is the way of moving from the description of the lived experience to the conceptualization of it in the language of science.

Essentially, then, the theory of Man-Living-Health, a formal theory described by Kaplan (1964), guides research and practice. The practice and research methodologies are presently evolving, and it is anticipated that the evolution and use of these methodologies will enhance the theory. The ontology and the congruent methodologies are offered as a contribution to the evolution of nursing science.

TABLE 11-4
Differences With Other Qualitative Research Methods

	Other Qualitative Methods	Man-Living-Health Method
Conceptual:	Phenomena are lived experiences	Entities for study are lived experiences–common experiences related to health as defined in Man-Living-Health
Methodological:	Retrospective descriptions, participant observation, and structured and unstructured interview are used to elicit descriptions from subjects	Researcher-participant dialogue elicits descriptions
	Analysis-synthesis moves data from concrete descriptions to abstract language of science	Extraction-synthesis moves participants' descriptions through conceptualizations by the researcher to syntheses of structures of lived experiences
Interpretive:	Hypotheses are generated through logical abstraction	Structures of lived experiences are created and theories are enhanced through heuristic interpretation

REFERENCES

Kaplan, A. (1964). *The conduct of inquiry.* Scranton, PA: Chandler Publishing Company.

Parse, R. R. (1981). *Man-living-health: A theory of nursing.* New York: John Wiley & Sons.

Parse, R. R., Coyne, A. B., and Smith, M. J. (1985). *Nursing research: Qualitative methods.* Bowie, MD: Brady Communications.

Rogers, M. E. (1970). *An introduction to the theoretical basis of nursing.* Philadelphia: F. A. Davis Co.

Rogers, M. E. (1980). "Nursing: A science of unitary man." In J. P. Riehl and C. Roy, eds. *Conceptual models for nursing practice.* 2nd ed., New York: Appleton-Century-Crofts. pp.329-337.

Sondheim, S. (1984) "Sunday." *From "Sunday in the park with George."* New York: RCA Records.
Tillich, P. (1952). *The courage to be.* New Haven: Yale University Press.

12

A Critique of Parse's Man-Living-Health Theory

JOHN R. PHILLIPS

Parse has developed a conceptual model that is unique to nursing. She did this by synthesizing Rogers's principles and concepts of the Science of Unitary Human Beings and the major tenets and concepts of existential-phenomenological thought. An explicit framework is provided that enables nurses to uncover the meaning of phenomena experienced by people. An understanding of the meaning of these phenomena—the lived experiences—also identifies the hallmarks of nursing: education, practice, and research.

Structure

HISTORICAL EVOLUTION

A variety of nursing models has been created in the past two decades. Many of these models draw on the traditional disciplines such as biology, medicine, physics, physiology, psychology, and sociology. The mechanistic view of Man is maintained in the majority of these models, where there is still a focus on particular parts of the person. Several of these models attempt to avoid this reductionistic perspective by summing all the parts to obtain what is assumed to be a holistic picture of individuals and their environments. In general, these models advocate the use of methodologies germane to the natural sciences, whereby quantitative data from observations are used to reveal causal relationships, which are considered pertinent to advancing nursing knowledge.

Considering the use of such models, one needs to be aware that one's view of reality is related to the conceptual model used to perceive the world. These mechanistic models have helped to perpetuate the idea that nursing does to or for people. Such a perspective conforms with Bush's (1979) idea that models enable persons to observe, order, clarify, and analyze events. However, Newman (1983) says "that what one sees or hears is only part of a greater reality. Intuition tells us that there is more there than meets the eye" (p. x).

Parse's scholarly work, *Man-Living-Health* (Parse, 1981), goes beyond the cause-and-effect and quantitative perspective of nursing science. Her model views nursing science as a process that holds its significance in dealing with the experiences of people. Such an approach enhances doing *with* people rather than to or for them. According to Parse, "Nursing, rooted in the human sciences, focuses on Man as a living unity and Man's qualitative participation with health experiences" (1981, p. 4). In order to present this humanistic perspective, Parse has synthesized the major ideas of Rogers's (1970, 1980) Science of Unitary Human Beings model with major tenets and concepts from existential-phenomenological thought to create her Man-Living-Health model of nursing, with the express purpose of understanding phenomena as humanly experienced. Parse's stance is supported by Donaldson's (1983) belief that "the value of scientific knowledge in nursing is determined by its relevance to and significance for an understanding of the human experience" (p. 41), with the express goal of helping people achieve health or wholeness. In addition, as early as 1973, Davis stated that "phenomenology provides a more perfect fit conceptually with the functions of clinical nursing and with many of the research questions that evolve from clinical practice" (p. 214). More recently, Fawcett (1984) implied the importance of a humanistic approach with her statement that "research derived from nurses' hunches about how to relate to clients is needed to validate observations and document the art of nursing and the therapeutic use of self" (p. 314).

However, Parse's model goes beyond Fawcett's research perspective to that of phenomenological research to understand human experiences from the perspective of the individual (Knaack, 1984, p. 108). Such a perspective no longer allows for perceptions that have been jaundiced by the natural sciences that encouraged nurses to view people as machines. In discussing phenomenology, Stevens (1979) pointed out "that no description of a phenomenon according to its components can fully explain the phenomenon . . . that experience and the thing to which it refers are inseparably linked" (p. 224). The lived experience deals with the wholeness of the person and negates the criticism that Parse does not deal with biological manifestations (Winkler, 1983, p. 289). Thus, Parse's model helps nurses transcend the parts' manifestations to lived experiences, the wholeness of the person. This is possible since Parse's (1981) nursing model is "a system of interrelated concepts describing unitary Man's interrelating with the environment while cocreating health" (p. 13).

With this in mind, it is easy to see why Parse chose to use Rogers's (1980) belief that a unitary human being and the environment are irreducible wholes. The synthesis of Rogers's model with the tenets and concepts of existential phenomenology is comprehensible when one accepts Stevens's (1979, p. 225) statement that existentialism, combined with the phenomenological method, enables the nurse to consider Man as a whole. In 1982 Limandri pointed out that "in combining Rogers with existentialism, Parse introduces an intriguing perspective of nursing phenomena that focuses on interrelatedness of humans to self, each other, and the environment" (p. 105).

Parse explicitly presents Rogers's principles of homeodynamics: helicy, resonancy, and complementarity (now called integrality), and the concepts of energy field, openness, pattern and organization (Rogers has recently deleted organization), and four-dimensionality (see Figure 12-1). The existential-phenomenological tenets of intentionality and human subjectivity and the concepts of coconstitution, coexistence, and situated freedom are presented equally clearly. It is obvious that Parse is cognizant of the need to be methodical in the elucidation of these principles, tenets, and concepts, since they serve as the basis for the creation of her Man-Living-Health model. Each is presented succinctly with the pertinent content needed for her model. An examination of the content reveals that it is accurate and consistent with the sources from which it was taken.

PHILOSOPHICAL ASSUMPTIONS

The importance of the explicit presentation of Rogers principles and concepts and the existential-phenomenological tenets and concepts becomes evident when the assumptions about Man and health are analyzed. This analysis makes it clear that these principles, tenets, and concepts were used to synthesize the assumptions. As stated by Parse (1981, p. 39), these assumptions underpin a view of nursing grounded in the human sciences. The reader does not have to hunt for the assumptions, or synthesize the content to determine what the assumptions are; they are stated in a straightforward manner (see Figure 12-1).

Parse uses the process of deduction to create each of the assumptions. Each assumption connects three specific concepts with one of the three concepts from Rogers and two from existential phenomenology or vice versa. This confirms that both Rogers and existential phenomenology are essential for the creation of each assumption. In addition, since each concept is related at least once with two others, each is necessary to the underpinning of the model. On further analysis of the relationship of the concepts in the assumptions, an interesting fact emerges that Parse does not address: two

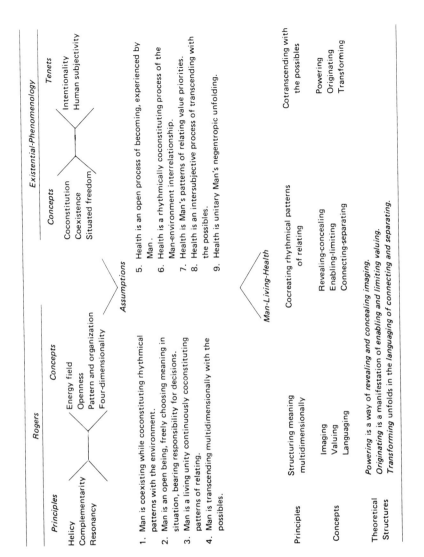

FIGURE 12-1
Evolution of the theory of Man-Living Health. (From Parse, R.R.: Man-Living-Health: A theory of nursing. New York, John Wiley & Sons, 1981, pp. 70-71.)

of the three concepts for each assumption come from Rogers for six of the nine assumptions, which leaves only three assumptions of which two of the three come from existential phenomenology.

PRINCIPLES, CONCEPTS, AND PROPOSITIONS

Although one may not agree with the content of Parse's model, one cannot fault her on the logic used to construct her model. Parse continues to use the deductive process to provide the structure through an explicit presentation of her three principles, nine concepts, and three theoretical structures. These components of her model emerge from the assumptions that were deduced from the principles, tenets, and concepts of Rogers and existential phenomenology. Each principle relates three concepts to each other (see Fig. 12-1), and a succinct description is given for each principle within the context of Rogers's Science of Unitary Human Beings model and the tenets and concepts of existential phenomenology. In addition, the use of pertinent literature further enhances one's ability to understand the connections of the three concepts. Furthermore, each concept is individually discussed in detail with extensive support from the literature. The final deductive elements of the structure of her model are the theoretical structures. The process by which these were deduced is discussed later in the correspondence section.

DEFINITION OF MAN

Man is one of the central concepts of Parse's model. Her views about Man pervade all elements of her model—assumptions, principles, concepts, and theoretical structures. Man is evident in all of the assumptions, and since the assumptions are used to construct her model, it is logical that Man should permeate throughout the structure of her model. Man is a living unity—"an experiencing subject who is more than and different from the sum of parts" (Parse, 1981, p. 177), a person who is characterized by pattern. Unitary Man interrelates with the environment while cocreating health. This is possible since Man coparticipates with the environment in creating becoming and is whole, open, and free to choose ways of living health. This is related to the fact that Man is an intentional being who is present with the world. This means interrelating with the various views of the world and others, and in fact participating in cocreating these views by a personal presence.

Thus, not only is Man involved in creating a personal becoming, but also as an emerging unitary phenomenon in the world with others. Being in the world with others, unitary Man participates in choosing personal situations and attitudes toward these situations. Man not only chooses meaning in the situation but also bears responsibility for decisions.

DEFINITION OF HEALTH

Health is another concept central to Parse's model that permeates all elements of the model. Health is not a static phenomenon in Parse's model, but a becoming process that is experienced multidimensionally by the person. It is an incarnation of Man's own choosing that is cocreated in the interchange of energy with environment. Thus, as Man and environment change rhythmically through connecting and separating, the phenomenon of health as a relative present is cocreated. In this sense, health is reflective of Man's way of living chosen, cherished ideals. Health is reaching beyond the actual through the process of transcending with the possibles. It is an emergent, negentropic unfolding. If health is transcending with the possibles, then it cannot be a linear concept deemed as good or bad, more or less, or even adapting or coping with the environment. Health is each person's own experience of valuing that can be known only through a personal description.

RELATIONSHIP BETWEEN MAN AND HEALTH

Parse's model is based on the view of science as a process. It provides a way of dealing with experience, a coming to know rather than being product-oriented. Since her model is grounded in the process of experiencing, the significance of the model title Man-Living-Health, becomes apparent. According to Parse (1981), "the hyphen demonstrates a conceptual bond among the words that creates a unity of meaning different from the individual words as they stand alone" (p. 39). Man lives and creates personal health through participation with the environment. This relationship is stated explicitly, with the fundamental tenet of the Parse model being that Man participates in health. This mutual relationship is manifest throughout the presentation of her model, and is depicted in the foregoing discussion of the definitions of Man and health. Again, it should be noted that the assumptions, which serve as the foundation of her model, deal specifically with Man and environment. Four of the assumptions speak directly about Man's relationships with the environment, essential to the living component of the model. The other five assumptions address health that is integral with the Man-environment relationship. Not only is Man a unitary phenomenon, but so is Man-Living-Health. The interconnected relationship of these concepts enables one to use methodologies to study Man's participative experiences in a situation, while participating in the creation of personal health.

Process

CORRESPONDENCE

Established Knowledge of Man and Health

There is a high degree of correspondence of Parse's model with general knowledge about Man and health. The established knowledge today about Man and health is moving more toward a unitary than a parts perspective. Parse's model utilizes this unitary perspective to provide a sound base for Man and health whereby it can be used for education, practice, and research.

Even though Parse presents a firm foundation for her perspective of health, there exists a body of knowledge, both before and after her model was created, that enhances the basis for her view of health. First, it should be noted again that Parse is not dealing with health that is related to particular parts of the person, but to manifestations of whole people as they interrelate with the environment. Parse's view of health goes beyond the reductionist view in which a "human being's knowledge, interest, abilities have become submerged" (Garrett and Garrett, 1982, p. 10). In getting away from this reductionist view, Dossey (1982, p. 148) showed how health involves all bodies since all bodies are involved in a dynamic relationship. Parse's transcendence of the parts enables a person to see that wounds produced by illness go far beyond the parts and "penetrate the existential depths of the person's being" (Curtin, 1979, p. 4). The significance of the dynamic relationship of the Man-Living-Health model is evident in Curtin's (1979) statement that "as we grow and mature we come to realize that although we are separate and distinct from all other creatures and the world, we belong to them and with them because we have grown out of the growth of others, learned from their knowledge and benefited from their suffering" (p. 3). Parse's view of going beyond the parts is also congruent with Winstead-Fry's (1980) belief that health transcends the physical and conveys the idea of meaningful interaction with the environment.

Health is a becoming process in Parse's model. Parse's idea that health is a becoming process is consistent with the belief of Bruhn and others (1977) that wellness is not a static state of being but rather a continuously evolving and changing process in which individuals participate. Does this not sound like Parse's view that Man cocreates health, where health is a manifestation of the unitary nature of Man-environment? Recently, Pepper (1985) pointed out that each person simultaneously experiences health as a process inclusive of strengths and weaknesses.

Health, according to Parse, is transcending with the possibles. Parse's concept of transcending with the possibles is reflected in the statement of Bruhn and others (1977) that Man is always surpassing what was once believed to be ultimate limits, a person's perception of potential is of significance to health. Parse's idea of obtaining the experience of the person in regard to health is inherent here and is also illustrated by Balog's (1982) view that health cannot really be known because it is neither an empirical fact nor an objective phenomenon. This is similar to Smith's (1981, 1983) idea—as well as Balog's idea (1982)—that health is a relative term.

Parse's concept of valuing is crucial to her postulations about health and is reflected in the view of Bruhn and others (1977) that wellness requires a person's action, decisions, and value judgments. In fact, Ferguson (1980, p. 248) has pointed out that health originates in an attitude: the acceptance of life's uncertainties, accepting responsibility for habits, a way of perceiving and dealing

with more satisfying human relationships, and a sense of purpose. In this respect, Moritz (1980, p. 54) sees health as a rhythmic
patterning of energy exchange that is mutually enhancing and expressing full life potential. Does this not encompass Parse's (1981)
assumption that "health is man's patterns of relating value priorities" (p. 25)? Parse (1984) also stated that "health is unitary man's
negentropic unfolding" (p. 25). Dunn (1977) also viewed wellness
as an orientation toward maximizing a person's potential. Too,
Smith's (1981, 1983) eudaemonistic model of health is concerned
with self-realization, the actualization or realization of one's potential—continuous growth and the refinement of sensibilities and
creativity.

It is interesting to note that the foregoing ideas of Parse about
health have been integrated into theoretical perspectives of holistic
health. Recently, Cmich (1984) presented theoretical perspectives
that postulate health as an expression of each person functioning
as a whole—an attitude as well as a lifestyle, a dynamic ongoing
process that reflects continuous change in the person's life, that all
are responsible for their own health, and that all are responsible
participants in creating health.

There is an established body of knowledge that views Man as
a whole, even though this perspective has not been reflected
throughout history, especially during the period of time when Man
was seen as a machine. Parse draws specifically from Rogers's
(1970, 1980) unitary human beings who are irreducible wholes—
more than and different from the sum of parts. Rogers (1970)
pointed out that the ancient Greeks saw "Man as a unified being
integral to the universe" (p. 43), and it is the perception of this
wholeness that will yield concepts and theories meaningful in
studying Man. Rogers, in providing theoretical support for her conceptualization of unitary human beings, has cited several persons
such as de Chardin (1965), Dubos (1975), and Polanyi (1958)—
the same individuals Parse cited in the creation of her model. However, there is further evidence that shows the fit of Parse's model
to established knowledge about Man.

Capra (1975) presented a theoretical perspective that shows
Man as a unitary person who is integral with the environment. It is
important to become aware that there is unity and mutual interrelatedness of all things, and to transcend the idea of the isolated

individual self. The essence of living systems can be understood only when the reductionist belief is abandoned (Capra, 1982, p. 108). Dossey (1982, pp. 148-149), in the presentation of a space-time model of birth, life, health, and death, used the unitary nature of human beings, the environment, and the dynamic interaction of the two. The body is not an object and cannot be localized in space. It has a dynamic relationship with all other bodies and with the universe.

Bohm (1980) pointed out that Man has always sensed that wholeness is a necessity to make life worth living. He (1980, p. 43) noted that Aristotle considered the universe as a whole whereby each part grows and develops in its relationship to the whole. Bohm (1980, p. 172) spoke of an enfolding-unfolding universe in which there is unbroken wholeness of the totality of existence with undivided flowing movement without borders. It was in this sense that Briggs and Peat (1984) stated that "the Chilean biologists say the identity of any living entity comes from its relationship with its environment" (p. 179). This dynamic process between Man and environment is present in Parse's assumptions, which serve as the ground for her model.

Parse's integration of the existential phenomenological tenets and concepts of intentionality, human subjectivity, coconstitution, coexistence, and situated freedom give further explication of the unitary nature of human beings and their dynamic mutual process with the environment. Unitary Man is characterized by patterns of relating that are coconstituted with the environment with the freedom to choose in the situation. Being an intentional, unitary human being, one is present and open to the world (Parse, 1981, pp. 18-21).

There is literature that supports this view other than that cited by Parse. Colodny (1982) noted that "the primary ontological position is that the world is an open one, the outcome of processes that are probabilistic in nature and constantly the domain of novelties and uncertainties" (p. ix). Colodny continued, "human thought moves always in quest of a unitary image of the world and towards a unified image of man" (p. xii). The noted Soviet scientist and scholar Nalimov (1982, p. 27) stated that evolution as a transformation should enable people to see changes in existing patterns as a whole being affected by another pattern—not as an additive process formed by ceaseless additions.

Interrelation of Concepts at Same Level
of Discourse

Once Parse constructed the assumptions for her model, she then focused on the creation of principles, concepts, and theoretical structures that can be used to describe, explain, or predict about Man and health. There are three principles, nine concepts, and three theoretical structures. Each principle interrelates three concepts (see Fig. 12-1).

Principle 1:
STRUCTURING MEANING MULTIDIMENSIONALLY IS COCREATING REALITY THROUGH THE LANGUAGING OF VALUING AND IMAGING.

The specific concepts for this principle are imaging, valuing, and languaging. This principle enables a person to cocreate reality by assigning meaning to multidimensional experiences that take place simultaneously in an infinite number of universes. The unique experiences are given form through personal languaging of imaging and valuing. According to Parse (1981), "weaving a 'fabric of meaning' in one's life, then, is structuring meaning multidimensionally through imaging, valuing and languaging" (p. 49).

Principle 2:
COCREATING RHYTHMICAL PATTERNS OF RELATING IS LIVING THE PARADOXICAL UNITY OF REVEALING-CONCEALING AND ENABLING-LIMITING WHILE CONNECTING-SEPARATING.

The essential concepts for this principle are: revealing-concealing, enabling-limiting, and connecting-separating. This principle means "there is an unfolding cadence of coconstituting ways of being with the world" (p. 50) through the rhythms of revealing-concealing, enabling-limiting, and connecting-separating. These rhythmic patterns can be seen in everyday life experiences as identifiable characteristics.

Principle 3:
COTRANSCENDING WITH THE POSSIBLES IS POWERING UNIQUE WAYS OF ORIGINATING IN THE PROCESS OF TRANSFORMING.

Powering, originating, and transforming are the specific concepts of this principle. This principle explains the power of original transformation through coconstituting with others. Man coconstitutes the situation and also cotranscends with it, thus living freely in situation within certain limits. Being free in situation Man can orient self toward the possibility by propeling self into future through powering and creating that which is beyond the self.

It is interesting to note how Parse created the theoretical structures from the three principles by using three concepts from the three principles. The three theoretical structures interrelate the three principles in a unique way such that one concept from each principle is used to create each of the three theoretical structures (see Fig. 12-1). This indicates each principle is necessary for the creation of each theoretical structure. Parse's (1981) three theoretical structures are:

1. *Powering* is a way of revealing and concealing imaging.

2. *Originating* is manifestation of enabling and limiting valuing.

3. *Transforming* unfolds in the languaging of connecting and separating. (p. 68)

One wonders, however, why the stem concept for each theoretical structure comes from the principle "Cotranscending with the possibles is powering unique ways of originating in the process of transforming" (p. 55). Without knowing the reason for this process, the writer speculates that greater importance might be attached to this principle, although Parse makes it clear that other theoretical structures may be generated from the principles of her model.

Relationship to Paradigmatic Perspectives and Philosophical Assumptions

Parse makes it clear that she is viewing science as a process that can be used in studying lived experiences. It is within the structure of science as sciencing that Parse (1981, pp. vii–x) has created her Man-Living-Health model to expand nursing science. Parse comes from two specific paradigms, Rogers's Science of Unitary Human Beings and existential phenomenological thought, predominantly Heidegger, Sartre, and Merleau-Ponty. Both of these paradigms deal with the unitary nature of Man and the universe— the becoming of Man through a dynamic relationship with the environment whereby Man is free to choose ways of living. Specifically, Parse has synthesized the identified principles, tenets, and concepts in building a model of interrelated concepts to describe how unitary Man creates health while interrelating with the environment. It is explicit how both of these paradigms are reflected in the assumptions of her model, as discussed in the above structure section. Writers have noted variations in focus on these two paradigms as Parse presents the principles, concepts, and theoretical structures, especially the concepts. Winkler (1983) noted "in Parse's elaboration of the meaning of the concepts that their derivation is primarily from the philosophical sources, and secondarily from Rogers [sic] model" (p. 281). However, it can be seen that each principle is couched within the perspective of the assumptions. And since each assumption is deduced from the two paradigms, it is logical to conclude that Rogers's work is inherent in the principles, concepts, and theoretical structures. Superficially, it may appear that the concepts for each principle come from existential phenomenological thought. However, as the complexity of the interrelationships between the concepts is grasped, it is apparent that Rogers's model serves as the basis for expressing the concepts and their interrelationships from an existential phenomenological perspective. This signifies the high level of abstaction Parse has achieved in making the two paradigms integral with each other. Within the science of nursing Parse's Man-Living-Health worldview evolves from the simultaneity paradigm (Parse and others, 1985).

Description and Meaning of Principles, Concepts, and Propositions

One unfamiliar with existential phenomenology may initially have difficulty with Parse's terminology. The terms have a process orientation as is indicated by the "ing" form for the principles, concepts, and the theoretical structures. This approach is consistent with the paradigmatic perspectives for the model, and it supports the unitary interrelatedness of Man, living, and health, as indicated by the use of the hyphen.

When looking at the major concepts of the structure of the model (for example, Man and health), one notes the presence of the same terms in their definitions, as well as in the assumptions, principles, and theoretical structure. Through this process, Parse is able to show the interconnectedness of her concepts, principles, and assumptions, and yet avoid circularity. As noted above, this enhances the process orientation of the model and builds on the paradigmatic perspective.

The cause-and-effect relationship is avoided through the creation of new terms such as cotranscending and cocreating to maintain consistency with the integral nature of Man-environment. A person does not create rhythmical patterns of relating, but these patterns emerge from the mutual creation by the person and the environment. This cocreating is given further specificity through the concepts of revealing-concealing, enabling-limiting, and connecting-separating. The meaning of such terms is made clear as each principle is described parsimoniously. It is through such succinct descriptions of each principle and its concepts that one gains the meaning of them, which enables one to understand each of the theoretical structures deduced from the principles. Understanding is further enhanced with the examples given and more recently with published compilation of research using her model (Parse and others, 1985).

Thus, when looking at the overall structure of Parse's model, one sees consistency in meaning at each level of discourse. The concepts in the assumptions present an abstract ground for the development of her model from specific paradigmatic perspectives. The principles and their concepts give greater specificity to this basis through which there is the genesis of the theoretical structures. It is these theoretical structures that nurses can concretize to provide the basis for education, practice and research.

COHERENCE

Relation of Theory to Other Theories

It is difficult to say definitely how Parse's principles are related to other theories. Briggs and Peat (1984, p. 24) have stated that theories or "paradigms" are like spectacles that people put on to solve "puzzles." A paradigm shift smashes these spectacles, and when new spectacles are put on, the world is viewed in a completely different way—whole new sets of puzzles can be seen. These authors specifically stated that "a new paradigm doesn't build on the paradigm it replaces; it turns in an entirely new direction" (1984, p. 31). In this sense, Zukav (1979) noted that:

Reality is what we take to be true.
What we take to be true is what we believe.
What we believe is based upon our perceptions.
What we perceive depends on what we look for.
What we look for depends on what we think.
What we think depends on what we perceive.
What we perceive determines what we take to be true.
What we take to be true is our reality. (p. 328)

Once Parse synthesized Rogers's and existential phenomenological thought, she created a new product, Man-Living-Health, a totally different way of perceiving reality. She is no longer speaking the exact same language as the sources from which she gained her new insight. Too, it is difficult to compare principles from various models that may be contradictory with one another. Fawcett (1984) also pointed out that "different models reflect different and logically incompatible views of the world" (p. 9). Thus, Parse's Man-Living-Health model, as expressed in her principles, no longer views Man as conceptualized by Rogers or existential phenomenological thought. Even Paterson and Zderad's (1976) work *Humanistic Nursing*, which draws from some of the same knowledge base of existential phenomenology, presents a view that is different from Parse's.

It can be seen, however, how Parse's principles are related to these two perspectives and to other nursing models. This is possible since there are presuppositions that surround her principles, which Fawcett (1984, p. 5) termed the metaparadigm of nursing—person, environment, health, and nursing. It is this metaparadigm that provides coherence of Parse's model to other nursing models, even though each model speaks a different language.

Parse's principles encompass the concept of the unitary nature of Man that is advocated by most of the nursing models. Parse's conceptualization of Man is most consistent, however, with Rogers where the whole person is perceived rather than the summative view of wholeness. In Parse's principles, unitary Man cocreates reality, cocreates rhythmical patterns of relating, and cotranscends with the environment. Even though all of the nursing models deal with the Man-environment relationship, Parse's principles are most consistent with Rogers's mutual process rather than the cause-effect or adaptation process manifest in other nursing models. One might say Parse's principles enable one to transcend the traditional view of nursing so phenomena can be explored in new ways to perceive the wholeness of Man through lived experiences. Ferguson (1980) stated that "when life becomes a process, the old distinctions between winning and losing, success and failure, fade away. Everything, even a negative outcome, has the potential to teach us and to further our quest" (p. 101). Parse's principles help one to see life as a process, a lived experience.

Logical Flow from Assumptions to Propositions

There is no question about the logic used in the construction of the Man-Living-Health model: the logical flow was indicated in the above structure section. Figure 12-1 gives a visual representation of the overall development of the model. To reiterate, as illustrated in the table, the principles, concepts, and tenets from Rogers and existential phenomenology were synthesized to create the assumptions for Man-Living-Health. These assumptions speak directly to the unitary nature of Man and of health as a process of becoming. These assumptions enabled Parse to postulate that Man-Living-Health is, itself, a unitary phenomenon. Three principles were then constructed to specify how Man lives health.

The three concepts for each of the principles were identified and discussed. Each of the three theoretical structures was then derived by using a concept from each of the three principles and showing the interrelationship of the concepts (see Fig. 12-1). Limandri (1982) stated "Parse very carefully, almost mechanistically, builds her theory" (p. 105): Parse used the deductive process in such a methodical manner to explicate her model so the reader would be able to understand each element of the model and how each element interrelates to create a whole—the ultimate goal being an understanding of the unity of Man-Living-Health as indicated by the use of the hyphen. Thus, the flow of the model moves from a highly abstract level to a less abstract one, as evidenced in the theoretical structures. It is the less abstract level that is discussed below in the pragmatics section.

Symmetry and Aesthetics

As one follows Parse in the explication of her model, one can feel her aesthetic sensations. The content is presented via structures that are pleasing to the eye and have a rhythmical flow as each element is built on the preceding one. One of the most pleasing aspects is the presentation of a schema that illustrates visually each element being developed. As elements are discussed, schemas are presented to illustrate how they interrelate with each other; these show how the elements are related symmetrically in an aesthetic way. The final schema shows the coherence of the complete model of Man-Living-Health.

PRAGMATICS

Use of Theory in Practice and Research

Parse has created an abstract model that can be used for education, practice, and research. Through the deductive process she has created theoretical structures that are less abstract and that can be used to generate research questions and to develop guidelines for practice. The empirical aspects are not as well developed as the structure of her model. However, Parse (1981, p. 78) pointed out that descriptive methodologies can be used to uncover a structure of meaning of lived experiences. Parse and others (1985) characterized such research approaches as a "study of Man's lived experiences in nonmeasurable terms" (p. 4). The descriptions by subjects can be used as data from which to identify and synthesize themes and common elements. The interpretation of the data describes the lived experiences and "generates hypothetical propositions through logical abstraction" (Parse and others, 1985, p. 4). Parse's theoretical structures enable identification of the characteristics of lived experiences and the significance of these experiences to those involved. Thus, the researcher is able to study emerging patterns of the Man-environment interrelationship, the person's participative experience in the situation being studied.

Parse's model is an abstract one from which innumerable research questions can be generated and investigated. These questions deal with the whole and not any one particular part of the person or family. In her book, Parse (1981) offered some lived experiences for study in relation to the theoretical structure. Two lived experiences with the related theoretical structures are:

Theoretical Structure:	Originating is a manifestation of enabling and limiting valuing.
Lived Experience	*Description*
Being enabled and limited by a choice	Describe a situation in which you experienced yourself making an important decision.
Being different from others	Describe a situation in which you experience yourself taking an unpopular stand on an issue. (Parse, 1981, p. 79)

One criticism of Parse's Man-Living-Health model has been that "in an attempt to relate her concepts she falls short of developing propositional statements that can be tested" (Limandri, 1982, p. 105). This criticism could be related to the fact that Parse calls

Man-Living-Health a theory, when in actuality it is a nursing model. Models supply a structure from which theories are generated. Bush (1979) and Lancaster and Lancaster (1981) have suggested that a model expresses structure while theory moves to the level of prediction to state relationships among components to provide substance in addition to structure. Parse's examples of phenomena that might be studied encourage persons to use their fertile imagination to create hypothetical propositions relevant to lived situations.

Parse has conducted several programs in which the results of research using Man-Living-Health have been presented. The literature reveals very little research using Parse's model, but it should be remembered that qualitative research is a time-consuming process, and once the research has been completed, it sometimes takes one or two years for it to be published. Parse's model was published in 1981, just four years ago. In April 1985, Parse and others published Nursing Research: Qualitative Methods. This publication presented research based on Man-Living-Health using several qualitative methods.

In the practice arena, the theoretical structures can be used to help people choose possibilities in their changing health processes. Winkler (1983, p. 292) pointed out that basing care planning on clients' perspective of health encourages nursing activities unique to the person. Parse presents in detail a family situation and how the theoretical structures can be used to illuminate patterns and mobilize energy toward the changing health perspectives evidenced by all members of the family.

There is an implicit guideline for practice in the Man-Living-Health model. In the discussion of the family situation, there is a presentation of the profile of a person from that perspective and from the perspective of all other family members. Basic to Parse's (1981) thesis is "Man's participation in and perspective of health as it is cocreated through interrelationships with others" (p. 82). The theoretical structures were used to illustrate how a nurse could participate in such situations "through illuminating patterns and mobilizing energies toward the changing health perspectives evident as the situation unfolded" (p. 83).

Recently Parse (1984) has developed guidelines regarding "Man-Living-Health in Practice" that specify the goal of nursing as quality of life as perceived from the person's perspective. The major section of the guidelines has specific questions that deal with (1) "Meaning—Thoughts and Feelings about Self and Situation," (2) Rhythmicity—Relationships with Others," and (3) "Transcendence—Dreams and Plans for Change (p. 1). The second section of the guidelines deals with the health profile from the person's and the nurse's perspective. There is also a section in the guidelines for the identification of emerging health patterns and activities. Concerning use of Parse's model in practice, she is currently serving as a theory consultant to a major health institution at which her theory is being tested.

Contribution to Nursing Science

Parse may well be one of the "Aquarian Conspirators" Ferguson (1984) wrote of who are involved in an enlarged concept of human potential. In addition, Leininger (1985) spoke of a movement that "calls for new ways of conceptualizing knowledge and experiences to discover the interrelatedness of diverse phenomena from a broad holistic and changing perspective" (p. 1). Parse certainly provides a conceptual model to help understand human phenomena and to stimulate the use of qualitative methods in creative ways to study lived experiences. According to Capra (1982), "Scientific theories can never provide a complete and definitive description of reality" (p. 48). Briggs and Peat (1984) have also pointed out that "for Einstein any theory based on statistics must be incomplete" (p. 75).

Parse's model will speed the transformation from a mechanistic approach to health care to one that has a unitary perspective of the health care of humans. Parse's model no longer allows for the interpretation of behavior from a parts perspective or determination by genetic makeup; there will be a focus on unitary Man-environment as Man creates health. People will better understand how Man chooses and bears responsibility for the rhythmical patterns of personal health. Parse's model will contribute to a transformation of the knowledge base of nursing and the practice of nursing from a unitary perspective. The Man-Living-Health model provides new hope that there will be greater focus in the future of the meaning and quality of life and health that transcends the disease orientation; it will deal with improved quality of life for all people as perceived by them.

Parse's use of unitary human beings, especially from Rogers and existential phenomenology that targets the pattern manifestations of the whole person, makes a contribution from a nursing science perspective to the emerging science of wholeness noted by Briggs and Peat (1984). Thus, Parse has not only used established knowledge about Man and health, her model also contributes to this knowledge.

REFERENCES

Balog, J. E. (1982). The concepts of health and disease: A relativistic perspective. *Health Values*, 6(5):7-13.

Bohm, D. (1980). *Wholeness and the implicate order*. London: Routledge & Kegan Paul.

Briggs, J. P., and Peat, F. D. (1984). *Looking glass universe: The emerging science of wholeness*. New York: Simon & Schuster.

Bruhn, J. G., Cordova, F. D., Williams, J. A., and Fuentes, R. G. (1977). The wellness process. *Journal of Community Health*, 2(3):209-221.

Bush, H. A. (1979). Models for nursing. *Advances in nursing science*, 1(2):13-21.

Capra, F. (1975). *The tao of physics*. Boulder, CO: Shambala.

Capra, F. (1982). *The turning point: Science, society, and the rising culture*. New York: Simon & Schuster.

Cmich, D. E. (1984). Theoretical perspectives of holistic health. *Journal of School Health*, 54(1):30-32.

Colodny, R. G. (1982). Foreword. *In* V. V. Nalimov, ed., *Realms of the unconscious: The enchanted frontier*. Philadelphia: ISI Press, pp. ix-xii.

Curtin, L. L. (1979). The nurse as advocate: A philosophical foundation for nursing. *Advances in Nursing Science*, 1((3):1-10.

Davis, A. J. (1973). The phenomenological approach in nursing research. *In* E. A. Garrison, ed., *Doctoral preparation for nurses . . . with emphasis on the psychiatric field*. San Francisco: University of California, pp. 213-228.

De Chardin, T. (1965). *The phenomenon of man*. New York: Paulist Press.

Donaldson, S. K. (1983). Let us not abandon the humanities. *Nursing Outlook*, 31(1):40-43.

Dossey, L. (1982). *Space, time and medicine*. Boulder, CO: Shambala.

Dubos, R. (1970). *Man adapting*. New Haven: Yale University Press.

Dunn, H. L. (1977). What high-level wellness means. *Health Values*, 1:9-16.

Fawcett, J. (1980). On research and the professionalization of nursing. *Nursing Forum*, 19(3):310-318.

Fawcett, J. (1984). *Analysis and evaluation of conceptual models of nursing.* Philadelphia: F. A. Davis and Co.

Ferguson, M. (1980). *The aquarian conspiracy: Personal and social transformation in the 1980s.* Los Angeles: J. P. Tarcher.

Garrett, S. S., and Garrett, B. (1982). Humaneness and health. *Topics in Clinical Nursing, 3*(4):7-12.

Knaack, P. (1984). Phenomenological research. *Western Journal of Nursing Research, 6*(1):107-114.

Lancaster, W., and Lancaster, J. (1981). Models and model building in nursing. *Advances in Nursing Science, 3*(3):33-42.

Leininger, M. M., ed. (1985). *Qualitative Research Methods in Nursing.* New York: Grune & Stratton.

Limandri, B. J. (1982). Book reviews. *Western Journal of Nursing Research, 4*(1):105-106.

Moritz, D. A. (1980). Nursing diagnoses in relation to nursing process. In M. J. Kim and D. A. Moritz, eds., *Classification of nursing diagnoses: Proceedings of the third and fourth national conferences.* New York: McGraw-Hill Book Co., pp. 53-58.

Nalimov, V. V. (1982). *Realms of the unconscious: The enchanted frontier.* Philadelphia: ISI Press.

Newman, M. A. (1983). Editorial. *Advances in Nursing Science, 5*(2):x-xi.

Parse, R. R. (1981). *Man-living-health: A theory of nursing.* New York: John Wiley & Sons.

Parse, R. R. (1984). *Man-living-health in practice.* Unpublished manuscript. Pittsburgh, PA. Discovery International, Inc.

Parse, R. R., Coyne, A. B., and Smith, M. J. (1985). *Nursing research: Qualitative methods.* Bowie, MD: Brady Communications.

Paterson, J., and Zderad, L. T. (1976). *Humanistic nursing.* New York: John Wiley & Sons.

Pepper, J. M. (1985, January/February). The wellness-illness continuum: Thoughts on changing nursing roles. *The Calendar,* pp. 6-8, 11.

Polanyi, M. (1958). *Personal knowledge.* Chicago: University of Chicago Press.

Rogers, M. E. (1970). *An introduction to the theoretical basis of nursing.* Philadelphia: F. A. Davis Co.

Rogers, M. E. (1980). Nursing: A science of unitary man. In J. P. Riehl and C. Roy, eds., *Conceptual models for nursing practice,* 2nd ed. New York: Appleton-Century-Crofts, pp. 329-337.

Smith, J. A. (1981). The idea of health: A philosophical inquiry. *Advances in Nursing Science, 3*(3):43-50.

Smith, J. A. (1983). *The idea of health: Implications for the nursing profession.* New York: Teachers College Press.

Stevens, B. J. (1979). *Nursing theory: Analysis, application, evaluation.* Boston: Little, Brown & Co.

Winkler, S. J. (1983). Parse's theory for nursing. In J. Fitzpatrick and A. Whall, eds., *Conceptual models of nursing: Analysis and application.* Bowie, MD: Brady Communications, pp. 275-294.

Winstead-Fry, P. (1980). The scientific method and its impact on holistic health. *Advances in Nursing Science*, 2(4):1-7.

Zukav, G. (1979). *The dancing wu li masters: An overview of the new physics.* New York: William Morrow.

Index

Note: Numbers in *italics* refer to figures.

205